"*Inarticulate Speech of the Heart* is filled with real and raw stories about human struggle and people facing adversity. With creativity, thoughtfulness, and humour, Larry uses these stories to explore how the beauty, complexity, pain, and longing of our experience points to a God who gives dignity, meaning, and purpose to life. This book is a satisfying meal for the soul!"

Christopher Barrett, national director, The Navigators of Canada

"An engaging, wise, funny, touching, probing, intelligent zinger of a book with the gift of grace. It seduces the reader with its powerful logic, sustained drive, and wonder. Perfection in so many ways."

Richard Taylor, writing instructor at Carleton University and author of
House Inside the Waves: Domesticity, Art and the Surfing Life

"This 'speech of the heart' is a compassionate inquiry into personal humanity and meaning following events, not unlike a lightning strike that changes the ground beneath. This experience resonates at a profound level that powerfully surpasses language and speaks to the endurance of the human spirit."

John Meissner, PhD, CPsych

LARRY J. MCCLOSKEY

Foreword by John Weston, Former MP

INARTICULATE
SPEECH
OF THE
Heart

Inarticulate Speech of the Heart
Copyright ©2021 Larry J. McCloskey

Published by Castle Quay Books
Burlington, Ontario, Canada and Jupiter, Florida, U.S.A.
416-573-3249 | info@castlequaybooks.com | www.castlequaybooks.com

Edited by Marina Hofman Willard.
Cover design and book interior by Burst Impressions.

Photo/art credits: Donald Menton (cover image), Cara Lipsett (Preface), Kristen McCloskey (Introduction, Chapter 12), Larry McCloskey (Chapters 4, 5, 10), Mike Nemesvary and Mark Junak (Chapter 9).

978-1-988928-39-5 soft cover
978-1-988928-40-1 e-book

Library and Archives Canada Cataloguing in Publication Data
Title: Inarticulate Speech of the Heart
Names: McCloskey, Larry J., 1955- author.
Identifiers: Canadiana 2020034725X | ISBN 9781988928395 (softcover)
Subjects: LCSH: People with disabilities—Biography. | LCSH: People with disabilities—Attitudes. | LCGFT: Biographies.
Classification: LCC HV1552.3 .M33 2020 | DDC 362.4092/2—dc23

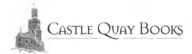

CASTLE QUAY BOOKS

Dedication

If work "is our love made visible" (Kahlil Gibran, *The Prophet*), it follows that the people you work with over the decades are the love of your life. This book is dedicated to the thousands of students and hundreds of staff I have had the privilege of working with these past 35 years. Most of all, this dedication is to my peeps from early days, too many of whom are no more.

*"Wisdom is the recovery of innocence
at the end of experience."*
David Bentley Hart, *The Experience of God:
Being, Consciousness, Bliss*

*"A human being is part of the whole, called by us the 'Universe,'
a part limited in time and space. He experiences himself, his
thoughts and feelings as something separate from the rest—a
kind of optical delusion of his consciousness. The striving to free
oneself from this delusion is the one issue of true religion. Not to
nourish the delusion but to try to overcome it is the way to
reach the attainable measure of peace of mind."*
Albert Einstein, winner of the 1921 Nobel Prize in Physics,
extract from a letter written to Robert Marcus, on the
passing of his son from polio (February 12, 1950)

A NOTE ON THE TITLE

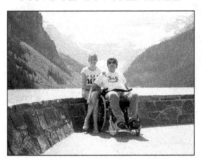

"Being human always points, and is directed, to something or someone,
other than oneself—be it a meaning to fulfill
or another human being to encounter."
Victor Frankl, writer, Holocaust survivor, psychiatrist (1905–1997)

One of Van Morrison's many great albums is entitled *Inarticulate Speech of the Heart*. Van attributed his arriving at this title to a Shavian (G. B. Shaw) saying, "of communicating with as little articulation as possible, at the same time being emotionally articulate." The title has always resonated with me because of the inarticulate nature of human existence.

For all the benefits of the modern world, people's inarticulate speech of the heart—that is, our inability to communicate the essence of who we are to those whom we want to be known by—seems a greater problem than ever before. I feel the problem in myself and decided to try to articulate something of my own pathetic speech of the heart throughout my years of taking care of, and being taken care of by, those whom God has placed on my path.

FOREWORD

By John Weston, Former MP, West Vancouver

I believe that someone asked to do a foreword for a book should like the book and know who the audience is that they are writing for.

On the first item, one can pick up any chapter in this book and know why I love every word of *Inarticulate Speech of the Heart*, for both its literary flourish and its deep wisdom. So, you can consider me an enthusiast.

As for the audience? If you're a parent or grandparent, Larry McCloskey's stories will help you translate today's turbulence into buckets of meaningful wisdom. If you're young, you'll receive a glimpse of the best and the brightest that your forebears had to offer. If you're able-bodied, you'll be challenged to do more with your gifts to help others. If you acknowledge your personal disabilities—and we all have them—you'll learn how challenges may reveal and then fortify your inner strength, your unique beauty, and your connection to your Maker. In short, anyone interested in life's meaning, who appreciates great storytelling, will enjoy and benefit from this book.

Larry's great writing is only one of the reasons to read his latest book, *Inarticulate Speech of the Heart*. The book is full of captivating stories that answer life's most difficult and important questions. One of his themes challenges us to record and quantify the gains and losses of our civilization as we evolved from the early twentieth century to the present. People born around the 1920s suffered through the Great Depression and fought World War II; they were "The Greatest Generation," as Tom Brokaw called them in a book by that name. They parented the baby boomers and, as grandparents, helped bring up Generation X and the millennials. Larry conveys reverence for their legacy through artistic yet frank glimpses of his own parents. He dovetails those observations with an assessment of the current human condition, earned through his unique work as a counsellor to people with disabilities. Marshalling these reflections, he positions us to examine our own condition—our own soul—to ask important questions of ourselves and our relationships and, as Tolstoy posed the question, "What must we then do?" He does all of this with memorable turns of phrase, vivid illustrations, and compelling prose.

Larry completed his book as COVID-19 consumed the world. For the first time in history, the whole world did something together: struggled with the uncertainty of a pandemic. Where do we go from here? Logical people have said that life will get more uncertain, not less. Larry grapples with questions that, more than ever, now engage us all.

What are you here for?

Is what you're doing worthwhile?

How do you measure your success?

How do you want to be remembered?

Who is your Maker?

What difference does it make?

What gives Larry the credentials to tackle such profound and compelling questions? Look no further than his germane experience that equipped him with countless relevant insights. His family life and circle of friends have seen tragedy. At the other end of the spectrum, he's enjoyed supreme achievement. In sport, Larry was a premier long-distance runner. Running enthusiasts will tell you not that he ran *well* (his form was notoriously bad) but that he ran *fast,* enduring pain, injury, and impediment, winning many tough races during a 30-year competitive career.

Speaking of impediments, Marcus Aurelius said, "What stands in the way … becomes the way." Whether you're buffeted by life's challenges or coddled from them, Larry moves you to realize that suffering forms character. The stretch realization is that character might even exceed happiness in importance. Larry lived that lesson long before Jordan Peterson achieved fame by writing about it.

Larry's work uniquely prepared him to talk about the soul. In serving quadriplegics, he learned what's left of human and transcendental value when a person loses control of most physical functions. As a former premier athlete, Larry was at one time focused on all the elements of physical prowess: exercise, nutrition, training, and equipment. What a revelation for someone immersed in physical achievement to work with people who lack the ability to move!

Another distinct thing about the book is the surreptitious nature of the issues Larry confronts. Like it or not, we don't naturally like to admit or talk about our disabilities. Yet we all have them. In fact, our capacity to acknowledge our disabilities allows us to examine what's really important about ourselves and about others.

For over 30 years, he has served as director of the Paul Menton Centre for Students with Disabilities at Carleton University, in Ottawa. Living in the capital has put him in touch with the pulse of a leading Western nation. In an Instagram world that pivots on people's superficial *strengths*, Larry has worked with thousands of young people to help manage their *weaknesses*, both perceived and real. Larry's perseverance in life and in vocation has provided him a front-row seat to observe the transformation of Western society.

These features—Larry's ability to persevere, his rich legacy of life lessons, his intricate latticework of human relationships, and his understanding of disabilities—

have prepared him to consider the soul. Something about Larry's life gets reflected in his book. He ran marathons for fun. He stuck with the same job for 30 years. He exemplifies "long obedience in a single direction," which Nietzsche said qualifies a person to live a life worth living.

One episode in the book is key to its understanding. The event in question relates to the photo that appears on the cover. Two brothers in 1976 take their quadriplegic third brother on a cross-Canada driving adventure, living out of the van along the way. When asked how the three of them traversed five thousand miles in close quarters while tending to the disabled brother's needs, one of them replied, "No big deal." As Larry writes, "*No big deal* was less a deflection than an expression of love … the inarticulate speech of their wounded hearts … Actions shout; words whisper."

In conclusion, if you love great writing, you'll love *Inarticulate Speech of the Heart*. If you care about the soul, you'll want to meet Larry. And, if you can't do that, you'll want to read his book.

PREFACE

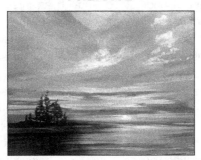

We are sponges—taking in, absorbing, filling up our whole lives, with love, with hatred, with experience, with an astonishing heap of life's minutiae that we can't necessarily take with us. But the means of accumulation is not material. The real purveyor of our heart's desire is the free-floating ride through time, space, abstraction, and human complexity into an infinity of possibility from our small finite lives.

We are far more than time travellers; we transcend the physical world through consciousness, the self-evident truth of our existence, including our innate ability to reason, interpret, and squirrel away experience into an evolving sense of self and, if we evolve, a fulsome sense of others.

Still, we are limited. We have a tragic flaw. We should star in a movie. For all our gifts and for all we accumulate, and for all we love or hate, and for all we time travel and transcend, we sure don't communicate much that matters. Especially to the people who matter.

Consciousness allows for astonishing connection between disparate parts—time, people, places—and being singular creatures, the interpretation of our life experience *must* be similar to other people's, and yet we don't personally know this to be true. Sadly, for most of us, the common denominator of human experience seems to be to live and die in a state of separateness. Consciousness has the potential to connect us to all things, except perhaps to each other.

Perversely, we seem to experience this non-experience without question. Knowing and seeing brilliant light from a star extinguished 10 million years ago is not only possible but easily accomplished after the setting of the sun. Expressing the inarticulate speech of the heart between one another remains fleeting to impossible.

The question is, why? Why are we not able to transcend the deep subjectivity of our heart's desire, the desire to be known? We explore the universe; we ignore the heart. The problem is not one of physiology. The physiology or mechanical functioning of the heart is understood, though an interesting anomaly to our understanding is the fact that for all we know—and by that, I mean from layperson to cardiologist—we do not really understand why it actually begins beating and continues to do so until we die. Understanding mechanism and understanding essence are two different things.

What emanates from the head is rational thought, whereas the heart is considered a deeper, more intuitive—even if murky—meaningful place. It may be that the notion of the heart has insight into who we really are, that our essence lies in the concept of the heart. Is the beating heart simply mechanical? Is the biology of humans simply cells that live and die, exist and are no more? Or is there more?

And if there is more—as science increasingly makes known—can more be incremental and contained, or is the admission of more a portal into the infinite? Can there be a short-term afterlife, a limit to loving, a small God? Is our resistance to acknowledge where consciousness leads us complacency, laziness, wilful blindness, or something else? Are we immobilized by the fear that there is nothing beyond the material world, or is the problem we sense beyond our senses a limitless explosion outside of the shallow known something of our everyday lives?

If there is no essence or soul, no experience will be recorded or arguably will have actually happened. What we call experience and what we feel is significant may be nothing more than highly sophisticated fraudulent brain function that has developed beyond its natural selection survival requirements, for no particular reason.

If there is no intention, *for no particular reason* becomes a convenient, trite way to explain away, well, everything. If you believe everything that happens in the world and in the universe is merely chaos somehow churning into workable unintended laws given a bit of time, good luck with that. Maybe better to contemplate the singularity of consciousness as the thing that sets us apart in the universe.

But we don't think about consciousness much, possibly because beyond taking it for granted, we avoid thinking as a defence against the ennui of modern times. That is, as creatures capable of deep insight we tend to avoid depth for convention to uphold the facade of normalcy and stay sane. Distraction is avoidance, with days passing without suffocating thoughts of oblivion seeping into every waking moment. Still, it is a mystery how people see a future for themselves and for their kids while figuratively standing in concrete shoes, petrified but compliant, slavish fodder for the oncoming freight train of life's inevitable end.

Faith's vacated space leaves a universe of space to fill. The new religion of materialism and atheism demands the denigration of God for good reason. Belief in God requires something of us, is not only about us, and goes against the tidal wave of modernity— individual choice at all times, fidelity to one's self first and foremost and to one's tribe as the main determinant to defining self. If our lifestyle choices are rituals and our individual selves sacred, then God is nothing more than *the* ultimate distraction that needs to be eliminated.

Progressive people profess to be atheists with this same predictable answer: *Logic is the currency of modernity, materialism, science, and technology, and God just ain't logical.* And I am ashamed to say, before I actually looked into the matter, my sense of wonder leading to a modicum of suspended faith was subverted by my failure to see the subversive and compelling logic of God.

The emerging consensus of our times about the non-existence of God bothered me, and not just because of the obvious reason that commitment to atheism is capitulation to death. I was bothered by that one little detail, my own ignorance. I wanted to investigate if my stubborn subjectivity—my hunger, my consciousness of being, my sense of wonder—was all I had to recommend myself, or if there might be objective ways to supplement or else erode conviction. I wanted to know if faith has any help. Turns out, as we muck around within material world limitations that we call our life, our greatest limitation is material-world thinking. The revelation of an examined life—in whatever circumstances we find ourselves—is that there is more, much more.

INTRODUCTION

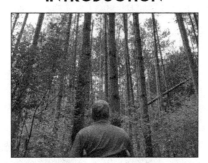

"Live life as if you were living a second time, and as though you had acted wrongly the first time."
Victor Frankl, writer, Holocaust survivor, psychiatrist (1905–1997)

As a grad student I got a job as an orderly for money. I chose to work on the spinal cord unit of the rehabilitation centre out of fear of immobility; same for long-distance running, though the reason for both was not apparent until years later. In the mix, I responded to a poster at the university asking for volunteers, but I wasn't needed. Instead, I ended up making a friend and getting his job. The part-time job became a full-time job, became the Paul Menton Centre for Students with Disabilities (PMC), became a place deeply immersed in *real*—real struggles, real challenges, real barriers, real people, real help mostly, and really frustrating always—and against intention and expectation became a vocation, a place to stay, home.

A place can only be home if there are people to share it. Our life's purpose may be as simple as how we greet those whom we meet—that is, what we do and who we are to whomever God places in our path—and for over 35 years my path has been filled by students with disabilities and staff at PMC (generically called disability service office, designated to provide student services and remove barriers in a university). My distance from wisdom and my accumulation of ignorance seem to have grown, but I have learned a couple things.

We need grit, are not wired for easy. You wouldn't know it in a world devoted to seeking comfort and distraction, but avoidance as a modern personal value isn't working out, is not going to save the world, is not good for those who populate this planet. Competing in distance running has helped to inform me. Training, getting stronger, faster, only happens from resistance, struggle, from committing to grit. Grit being the counterintuitive equivalent to eating our pound of dirt in order to have a healthy immune system. We do not need, it does not help us, to get everything we want, desire, and possibly deserve or to realize our heart's desire unless it is to be known.

Personal goals are fine, but they will not liberate, will not elevate us to our higher selves. We need goals and outcomes to be shared to have meaning, to bring together our splintered physical, psychological, and spiritual selves. "I am struck by how sharing our weakness and difficulties is more nourishing to others than sharing our qualities and successes" (Jean Vanier).

Turns out, altruism and self-interest can be the same, along the same shared path, which can be our life's work. In my work at PMC, I have received more than I have given, for which I am grateful in perpetuity. Though decades in the making, most of all I am grateful to have learned that work "is our love made visible" (Kahlil Gibran, *The Prophet*).

Everything we do our whole life is an attempt to break free and articulate our heart's desire. Much of life is struggling to find some equilibrium within circumstances that are beyond our control and our ability to even comprehend. For all modernity's emphasis on individual choice, we are bandied about by the vicissitudes of life and, on balance, pull off living the cards we are dealt pretty well. Life is hard, and it is easy to feel unworthy or resentful and simply give up and submit to addiction, distraction, and the blandness of it all. Still, the profound and uplifting reality is that we get up and live to fight another day.

The people in my personal account might be regarded as common or unexceptional by modern celebrity culture, but to the examined mind, their lives are quite astonishing. Most have endured tragedy or hardship and may seem to have lived compromised lives, but that would be to miss the point of this book. Enduring tragedy and living a tragic life are not the same, nor even necessarily related.

The most spectacular lives, those lives that can instruct us best on how to live life well regardless of circumstance, tend to pass unnoticed by the distracted majority. The difference between mundane and miracle—a spiritual truth as well as a proven theorem in quantum mechanics—is related to and affected by the eye of the observer.

This book is an attempt to articulate something of the inarticulate speech of their wounded, perfect hearts. I want the people of my path to be known, I want to be known, so I articulated the following account.

Chapter One

WHERE HAVE ALL THE YOUNG QUADS GONE?

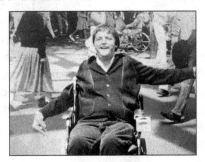

"If there is meaning in life at all, then there must be a meaning in suffering. Suffering is an ineradicable part of life, even as fate and death. Without suffering and death, human life cannot be complete."

Victor Frankl, writer, Holocaust survivor, psychologist (1905–1997)

In the first five minutes of my first shift I was ordered to perform a "digital." A digital is part of the regular routine for a quadriplegic. It is done every few days by an attendant because the paralysis from permanent, traumatic spinal cord injury extends to the ability to s**t. Voluntary physical function below the level of injury is either compromised or more likely no longer possible. Both bowel and bladder control are affected, as well as the ability to feel—anything. Well, not exactly true; quadriplegics feel intensely the pain of being unable to feel.

The digital routine is unpleasant to perform and is humiliating to have to submit to. And the stark reality for those who sustain high-level spinal cord injury is that the digital is but one of several daily indignities that have to be endured. Worse still, the digital does not necessarily top the list.

My first patient's name was Chris. He had been injured for just six weeks. Chris had spent the previous weeks stabilizing at the Ottawa Civic Hospital before being transferred to the spinal cord unit of the rehabilitation centre, then a single floor of a psychiatric hospital. Chris and I did not know each other. We were not introduced before I began the necessary procedure.

A young guy who had roared down country lanes on his motorcycle in the liberating spring after a Canadian winter lay imprisoned in a room with three other spinal cord patients, windows shut to keep summer from seeping in, with a novice unwanted stranger doing unwanted strange procedures, who would stroll away in carefree fashion at the end of his shift. In the meantime, one-way small talk while sticking my finger up his a*s, pulling the contents of his bowels onto a waiting diaper, and trying to ignore the odour. Life had come to this. Thoughts of death clustered in gathering clouds too vague, painful, and confused to act on.

The digital may have been my saving grace, as in, if you can survive the first half hour, the rest of the shift is relatively easy. So I thought. I was given a full workload, that my first day. The workload was heavy—not just busy but literally heavy. The morning routine for a quadriplegic is slow and demanding and requires patience (a virtue alien to me but not to the people I worked with), since providing intimate care to reluctant recipients is highly variable according to individual differences, if patients do not lose their humanity during the indoctrination of routine.

A quadriplegic is paralyzed in all four limbs compared to a paraplegic's two, the former spinal breakage at the neck, the latter the back. Seems fairly straightforward, and yet the terms are often interchanged as if the same thing. They are not. Quadriplegia is a much more difficult condition, with far greater limitations to contend with.

Paraplegics manually propel their own lightweight wheelchairs; have bowel, bladder, and sexual function; transfer themselves; and otherwise live independent lives. Quadriplegics likely require lifetime personal attendants; may need to be turned at night to prevent bedsores; may need assistance eating, dressing, and transferring; and for mobility they use an electric wheelchair, sometimes operated by head movements if the injury is high enough on the spinal column.

Quadriplegics are difficult to turn, move, and transfer and, given an enforced life of inactivity, are prone to put on weight, to add insult to spinal cord injury. Peter, the much older, seasoned orderly who was to show me the ropes, was much occupied with his own patients, so I relied on my four new friends for edification, they lying in bed waiting for me to figure out how to accomplish the impossible.

Once the morning routine was done, there were various therapies to get to— part of the therapeutic strategy being to inspire purpose by being busy, I guess. (In at least one case I know that this strategy worked out far beyond expectations. A young guy, isolated and severely depressed, jumps from a five-storey building, it not being high enough to kill him but of sufficient height to inflict permanent spinal cord injury. He wakes up in hospital smothered in therapists, has people to see and places to go, and regains a sense of purpose. It should be noted that his response to the rehab gig is spectacularly exceptional and not to be followed.)

The list of professionals whose lifetime ambition is to poke and prod is long— occupational therapists, physiotherapists, social workers, and psychologists, among others. Which is not to disparage rehabilitation professionals. They do good, important work, but professionalism is far from the minds of recently injured patients, for whom indoctrination can feel deeply intrusive.

Getting to therapy involved transferring to a wheelchair, and I had no idea how to do it, that it could be done. I waited looking for someone, anyone, to ask, but there was no one, only my four friends waiting for transfers to be able to get on with their appointments. I didn't know what to do—theme of the day—and quickly concluded that I would just have to find a way to do it—second theme of the day as a result of the first.

My guys were heavy, quadriplegia being the definition of dead weight. Getting from bed to wheelchair required what was called a two-man transfer, basically one person lifting from behind under the arms and gripping the chest area, and the other facing the front and lifting the legs above the knees. Finally, Peter passes by and tells me without stopping that the thing is, there are rarely two men available, so you just have to learn how to do a one-man transfer. That simple.

He felt sorry for me and condescended to give me a 30-second demo. Electric bed up into sitting position—better do it slowly because if you go too fast your patient will faint; pull person up farther and rotate legs so that they hang over the bed, pointing to the floor; important keystone piece here for the architecture of your maneuver is this: lock your knees outside said patient's knees, bend over and place your arms under his pits, then lean back, way back, for ballast, and pull him into a very temporary standing position. (Peter didn't say it, but I soon incorporated prayer into this critical step of the maneuver.) Now pivot and aim for the wheelchair and let go, slowly; oh yeah, and don't forget to put the brakes on the chair, or else your guy will end up flat on his back with you on top. Which wouldn't be good, but hey, at least we wouldn't be risking spinal cord injury, my guys would deadpan.

After this instruction, who wouldn't have confidence doing a one-man (me at 135 pounds) transfer of 270 pounds of a recently injured and, in spite of patients' cavalier double jeopardy joke, highly vulnerable quadriplegic human being? In retrospect, I don't remember being overly stressed after doing my first transfer, though each one was challenging and required every bit of strength and concentration I had. More amazing was that the guys I worked with—adventurers who had paid a deadweight heavy price—allowed and even encouraged me, half the man that I was. If I managed to suppress feelings of stress, these guys were uniformly calm, jocular even, as we danced and pivoted from bed to chair, always one percent away from disaster, but me never actually dropping anyone. I doubt the one-man transfer remains a rehab centre staple anymore, at least as performed by scrawny staff dis-orderlies exactly half the weight of the brave patients.

I was given no training on that my first day, same for every other. Still, I wasn't thrown to the wolves. My newly injured patients were patient, and together we joked, giggled, and problem-solved until the job was done. Though I was called an orderly, much of the work I did then has been taken over by nurses, with four-year university degrees as a minimum. And some of the procedures we orderlies routinely were assigned to do and did without question then now require a medical specialist. This was 1980, before the age of regulation, for better or worse.

It is fair to say that I absorbed more of value in my first shift as an orderly on that spinal cord unit than I learned during two completed university graduate programs, the content of both degrees an irrelevant blur, whereas every frame of every scene and every person in it on the spinal cord ward still hangs in my personal gallery of valuable experience and will remain there for life. It is because of my work as an orderly that I continued from a master of arts to a master's degree in social work. That degree required doing a three-month placement in the same rehab hospital that I worked in as an orderly.

But the clinical placement was disappointing compared to the ongoing dialogue of an orderly shift. The clinical placement had formal scheduled appointments that involved asking people how they felt while offering nothing to help alleviate how they felt. But as an orderly I could steal in at 3 a.m. to turn a patient from one side to the other, who being awake and without being asked how he felt might divulge deepest feelings just 'cause. Or to put a finer point on it, while doing something useful, and without soliciting for feelings, I was willing to listen and could be trusted.

Hands-on work in the service of others, even or especially if said task is a bowel routine, has more value than most of contemporary formal education. No thinking (thank God), no agenda, no theorizing, no virtue signalling, just doing; useful, and not about self, the abnegation of self accomplished by the completion of a task in spite of the smell. Extension of the metaphor—much of life is s**t; a life well lived is what we do about it.

Back to my first task with my first patient on my first day. On the giving end of the digital, I did not feel disgust. Maybe I felt something akin to self-disgust for what I had to do to Chris, exposed like a putrid frog about to be dissected by pimply high school students eager to mutilate and maim designated deadness. Exposure day and night for remaining days and nights. At least these are thoughts, impressions, from some whose sense of drowning in the early days is supplanted by the possibility of a life treading water.

It takes a long time to accept or even comprehend the incomprehensible loss due to severe spinal cord injury. Waking each morning is to be consigned to a nightmare from which there is no waking. Six weeks being injured had not convinced Chris to capitulate to the inevitable. He had more fight in him than that. He had been a risk-taker and a rebel and was not about to reconcile himself to the conventions of bladder care and pressure sore prevention. Waking into screaming morning light and the nightmare of immobility from repeat rebellious dreams of glorious movement, he flailed atrophying fists into dead legs as best he could, willing the sensation from that which cannot feel. Physical pain would have afforded welcome relief.

Daily daytime nightmare confirmed and anger vented, he exited rage and reverted to an unfeeling state of mind to match his unfeeling lower body. His roommates didn't exist; if you were in the room he didn't see you. I never saw him look outside his window; he didn't see summer; he never seemed to look at anything. His unseeing extended to the truncated life that was to be his future.

All happy experiences are alike; each unhappy experience is unhappy in its own way. Yes, my sentence blatantly steals from Tolstoy's famous opening to *Anna Karenina*, with slight alteration. Still, universal truths can lend themselves to such blatant appropriation. Happiness is most often involved with shared experience; people generally suffer alone, suffer more as a consequence of isolation than of circumstance, the exile of inarticulation that is the human condition. Still, for all the pain, there are poignant moments that sear the banal with the hint of possibility, proof of shared consciousness even from unlikely sources.

Jim was a big rangy guy, recently back to the rehab centre from a Texas hospital after a failed life-saving treatment for a rare vascular congenital condition. He was a guy's guy, had worked at the GM factory in Oshawa, was now a quadriplegic, was soon going to die. Though he didn't have much time, he had lots of visitors. All big guys, all auto workers, all awkward and caring, lots of standing around, four or five huddled around Jim's bed, little said, volumes in the gaps that are the poignant hum of communal silence.

Sports, their bar back home, well-trodden jocular barbs, someone's old girlfriend recently spotted, how long they had all hung together, covered the range of discussion. Nothing about Jim's condition or where his condition was taking him, especially from Jim. Hulking killers if they wanted to be, gentle as puppies as I brushed by to fill Jim's water bottle or empty his leg bag. For hours they stood, either unable to leave or not knowing how. Remarkably, they didn't just make a single requisite visit; they came back often, driving long hours in their company-discounted GM trucks to see Jim.

And for all their muted articulation, something imperceptible seemed to pass between these odd exemplars of connection by way of few words and humble gestures. Later one evening, as four guys silently drove home to Oshawa, I crept back to check on Jim. Checking on Jim never involved inane talk, just a word or two and a brief ghost-like presence, doing something if something could be done and leaving if not.

But on this one solitary occasion, Jim suddenly, quietly, spoke a few heartfelt words to my exiting inarticulate backside. "If I'd had a brother, I'd have wanted him to be like you." I stopped and smiled but didn't, couldn't, answer. I owe Jim, even if acknowledgement comes decades late and with far less grace than his mostly silent, ever vigilant friends.

Five minutes into my next shift a nurse touched my arm and told me Jim had died. I went to his room and stood where I had been when we had last spoken—that is, his heartfelt words and my inability to give him the same. The room and my failure to speak echoed as empty as the cosmos.

Chris's experience was absolutely unique, but his reaction to the cataclysm that had descended upon him had a certain familiarity I was about to see among other young, once spirited, men: anger, outrage, a deep sad sense of bewilderment, followed by an involuntary emotional retentiveness, retreating into a dark, inaccessible place. As the days progressed, as I invisibly performed my utilitarian function, I wondered about Chris's story, all their stories, and how in the world they could ever make their way through such a cruel plot line. But this wasn't fiction, just stranger than fiction. This was life, each individual's personal one-and-only life.

I'd like to say that in my compassion, I spent much time pondering Chris's story, even if I couldn't change it. But the claim would be disingenuous. We were busy, and much as we tried to become more efficient, it was always chaotic. We were chronically understaffed, and the exacting human nature of our work meant that factory-like efficiency was never going to happen. Which, at least in part, is what attracted me to this line of work. I liked the people, and for all their trauma, they retained and, more often than not, grew in their humanity. Which is not to say that their accident, their trauma, their struggle was a good thing. Only someone patronizing and detached from the experience would say that. I am not saying that. Still, for all the physical torture, there was palpable spiritual growth for some. And for the others, not so palpable, but growth nonetheless.

In fiction, the narrative necessitates struggle, tension being relieved by the protagonist who overcomes the struggle and finds resolution, and with the narrative arch complete, the audience is left passively satisfied. Quadriplegics struggle mightily, and many create and manage to live productive lives, in time. Incredibly, many manage to pull an actual life from the embers of a life destroyed, but they do not overcome struggle, just adversity. The many therapies do not instruct broken people on how to become whole again, and although the word is overused, it is fully applicable here: people *courageously* work it out for themselves.

I have seen people work out for themselves a version of higher self, beyond physical world adaptation, though my understanding is far from complete. The problem is, the twin pillars of atheism and scientific materialism have become modernity's substitutes for the archetypal and self-evident truth of spiritual life.

Atheism reduces human life to temporary cellular function, for which meaning is not examined and purpose is the avoidance of pain. The stripping of *what was* for the emptiness of *what is* requires context, examination, and, my radical thought is, the application of critical thought. The value of Chris and the meaning of what happened to him hang in the balance.

Perhaps no one encapsulates the assault upon what *was* for the epoch of what *is* more than Richard Dawkins. *The God Delusion* is considered by his many millions of adherents as a tour de force, daring to disparage organized religion for its subjugation of individual freedoms and human rights. As a renowned scientist—he is an Oxford biologist—his use of science and logic are considered a breath of fresh air blowing away the cobwebs of superstition and archaic meaningless ritual.

I tried to read *The God Delusion* with an open mind. Reader alert: I may have failed in this endeavour. My lack of objectivity may have been influenced by a documentary I saw on Netflix just as I began reading the book. The film was an atheist dreamlike concert tour featuring Dr. Richard Dawkins and Dr. Lawrence Krause, a physicist, whose own seminal work *A Universe from Nothing* made these two the perfect celebrity team, together exposing both the creation of the universe and the beginning of life on earth as wholly material events wherein God was not required.

What is striking about the documentary is this: even if the facts and logic support their atheist premise, what could possibly account for the cult-like reception from tens of thousands of adoring fans to what amounts to—however gloriously packaged—inevitable oblivion of that very personhood to which atheism and materialism are devoted? What could possibly motivate people to flock to the great articulators of nothingness?

In *The God Delusion* (Dawkins's magnum opus, bolstered by another 15 books), the good doctor employs an adept understanding of the psychology of his enthusiastic audience. In the modern material world there is nothing more valuable than the illusion of endless personal choice and nothing more threatening than its opposite. It is no wonder that Dawkins's audience loves his message since even the meaning of the central theistic religions is perceived as opposition to the sanctity of the individual—*Catholic* means "universal," *Islam* means "surrender," and *Judaism* means "thank you" or "gratitude." No individual choice or self-expression here.

Dawkins understands and appeals to people's sense of victimhood—assumes this to be a steady state—for what they have suffered at the hands of religion. A minor omission may be that his argument does not attempt to compensate for inevitable oblivion, but hey, that's only when the party ends, and who knows, science may have naturally selected them for eternal life by then.

Though Dr. Dawkins regards science and logic as irreconcilable with religion or belief in God, science is hardly straightforward or without contradiction. For example, as far back as the 1920s, emerging quantum mechanics revealed that light can behave as either a particle or a wave. And what accounts for this difference in behaviour? To the surprise of scientists then, and to everyone's continued puzzlement 100 years later, the answer is that light and matter only behave as particles when in the presence of an *intelligent observer*. Equally fantastical is the Heisenberg uncertainty principle, which revealed that one can measure either the position or momentum of particles but not both at once. Doesn't make sense, I know, but nonsensical as it is, for all these decades it has been often proven and universally accepted by physicists as true.

Quantum mechanics has many astonishing anomalies and has been described by many as quantum weirdness. In a very real sense, atoms and molecules lack reality and exist as potentiality until observed—a phenomenon about which Einstein famously remarked, "I like to think the moon is there even when I'm not looking at it." What is implied in Einstein's facetious remark is that there is no reason to assume that the weirdness of quantum mechanics only happens on the microscopic level.

Echoing Einstein recently without a hint of facetiousness, Amit Goswami, an accomplished quantum physicist, wrote, "There is no object in space-time without a conscious subject looking at it." Goswami questions our fundamental material-world assumptions, the very nature of reality, on the basis of science and concludes that the existence of God needn't only be a matter of faith.

Perhaps nothing about quantum mechanics shakes our perceptions about material-world reality more than the concept of *entanglement*, which occurs when a pair or group of particles interact or share proximity. In the 1930s, quantum physicists mathematically proved, and later demonstrated, that entangled particles can communicate faster than the speed of light, likely instantaneously, regardless of distance between split/entangled particles. According to Einstein's universally accepted theory of relativity, nothing can travel faster than the speed of light, and yet entanglement proves otherwise, leading to the mind-blowing concept of *non-locality*, which implies a universe wherein distance does not exist.

The implications of entanglement leading to non-locality cannot be understated. The physical world as we perceive it is not real as proven by science, and therefore another realm logically exists beyond our senses but not necessarily outside of our consciousness. In *The Physics of God* Joseph Selbie makes a superb case that challenges scientific materialism with an argument for spiritual potential based on science. People commonly say *science is settled* as a means to limit discussion about an issue they have settled on regardless of science. But in the interests of openness and continued discovery, science is never settled. To that end, Selbie cites physicist Nick Herbert: "One of the best-kept secrets of science is that physicists have lost their grip on reality."[1] And that is the good news. Science needn't be settled to arrive at an interpretation that God and science are entangled.

Which challenges the great divide in Dawkins's mind: science and reason versus religion and superstition. It never seems to occur to him that science and spirituality might not be mutually exclusive, that there might be a logic to God, not only in consideration of science but especially as a result of having studied where our knowledge of science logically leads to and where knowable scientific materialism ends. Though scientific materialism steals the headlines today, far less well-known are those many scientists whose views converge on this single simple premise: *the logic of science does not necessarily lead to logical interpretations of its findings.*

A non-biased logical reconciliation of science and spiritually is the stated purpose of renowned scientist Dr. Francis Collins in *The Language of God*: "belief in God can be an entirely rational choice, and that the principles of faith are, in fact, complementary with the principles of science."[2] I read his book when I began my odyssey out of ignorance and so recognized his name in a *National Post* article by Sean Speer in July 2020 about "one of the most important people in the world."

1. Joseph Selbie, *The Physics of God: Unifying Quantum Physics, Consciousness, M-Theory, Heaven, Neuroscience and Transcendence* (Newburyport: New Page Books, 2018), 30.
2. Francis S. Collins, *The Language of God: A Scientist Presents Evidence for Belief* (New York: Free Press, 2007), 3.

Dr. Collins, a physician-geneticist, was the lead scientist of the Human Genome Project, which mapped the full sequence of three billion DNA letters of the human blueprint. This project, taking 13 years and costing three billion dollars, is possibly the greatest coordinated scientific achievement of all time. Recently, as head of the National Institutes of Health, Collins coordinated a massive project involving 18 pharmaceutical companies and government agencies working for a COVID vaccine. Still, for all his qualifications, Dr. Collins recognizes the need to expand one's thinking beyond science in consideration of the big questions, citing the final paragraph in astrophysicist Robert Jastrow's *God and the Astronomers*:

> At this moment it seems that science will never be able to raise the curtain on the mystery of creation. For the scientist who has lived by his faith in the power of reason, the story ends like a bad dream. He has scaled the mountains of ignorance; he is about to conquer the highest peak; as he pulls himself over the final rock, he is greeted by a band of theologians who have been sitting there for centuries.[3]

I am my father's son. My father, a self-described maverick, taught me to exercise healthy skepticism—that is, to not accept as fact what does not pass the smell test. I contend that there exists a world of logic informed by gut feeling (common sense, combined with the practice of becoming informed before voicing opinion, and willingness to be wrong) that is not limited by science. I mention this just before delving back into Dawkins's scientific explanation of all things because I suspect we spend most of our lives explaining away the few and fleeting self-evident truths that we experience for lack of confidence, for fear of offending the progressives of these intolerant modern times. Repression is not liberating and silence is not golden, but they help explain the inarticulate speech of the yearning heart.

Dawkins's explanation of the origin of the universe is an interesting exercise in free-range interpretation. It is worth mentioning that throughout the twentieth century there were huge scientific breakthroughs proving the origin of the universe to be what is now known as the big bang. Perhaps most notable, and a tad ironic, is the fact that the father of what was to became known as the big bang theory—the scientific breakthrough of all time—was a Belgium Roman Catholic priest, physicist, and astronomer—Georges Lemaitre.

In 1929, he is credited with the first definitive formulation of an expanding rather than static universe. Interestingly, in 1931, at a meeting in London to discuss the relationship between the physical universe and spirituality (before such discussion became so uncool), Lemaitre proposed that the universe expanded from a single point, which he called the "primeval atom" or "cosmic egg," which exploded at the moment of creation. This moment, originally called *singularity*, was later changed to *the big bang* based on a sarcastic comment made by astronomer Fred Hoyle

3. R. Jastrow, *God and the Astronomers* (New York: W.W. Norton, 1992), 107.

in 1949. Initially, Einstein responded to Lemaitre's theory with the comment, "Your math is correct, but your physics is abominable." However, by 1933, his theory had gained widespread support in the scientific community, and after hearing Lemaitre, Einstein is reputed to have said that "this is the most beautiful and satisfactory explanation of creation to which I have ever listened."

There are some, Dawkins among them, who regard the big bang as a victory for science, since the big bang was irrefutably a scientific event. But what should be troubling for atheists and scientists alike is that the big bang proves the universe is not infinite but came into being at a defined moment and therefore requires an explanation of origin—that is, it raises the question, What preceded the big bang?

There is no provable explanation for what caused the big bang, though Dawkins offers the feeble theory of endless regression—that is, endless expansion and shrinking of the universe, perpetual big bangs—which is a wild theory that cannot be proven and really has no basis in science. He further speculates on the existence of a "multiverse," again continuing on the infinity schtick, which again conveniently allows for faux-scientific theory without scientific basis, but with just enough of a sniff of science fiction to shock and awe with possibility.

As Dawkins postulates the multiverse theory, he does concede that there may be "gaps" in his thesis, before insisting that the existence of God is *the bigger problem*. Particularly for a scientist, this argument is disingenuous because the discounting of one problem does not prove the other. And of course, if you refuse to consider the possibility of the existence of God before beginning your scientific enquiry—thereby eliminating the scientific objectivity essential to scientific enquiry—you are left with Dawkins's oft used explanation that *science will fully explain everything when we get to it,* thus making an implausible "gap" argument into a compelling and sexy theory. Not very satisfyingly, and betraying the basic principle of causality. Endless regression of the big bang does not explain origin, is really only a theory of avoidance. There has to be an original cause of the big bang, or even big bangs; otherwise one is making a circular, not a scientific, argument. To be clear, there is absolutely no evidence to support repeated big bangs or a multiverse theory, and thus they are science fiction, given dubious credibility by the reputation of the popular author, coupled with the receptivity of well-educated audiences in these gullible, progressive times.

Dr. Dawkins is unwilling to consider the possibility that God *is* the infamous gap that balances and complements science, even as Dr. Collins and an increasing cadre of reputable scientists have become convinced on the basis of empirical evidence. His fundamental contention is that science, and science alone, will explain all things once it gets to it. Time and the elimination of ignorance—religion—will allow for the total explanation of everything.

Interestingly, scientific materialists often invoke the larger than life figure of Stephen Hawking to support their arguments. Throughout his writings, Hawking's arguments are more aligned with atheism than not, but he is not entirely consistent. Or perhaps he recognizes the inevitability of contradiction when a scientist must concede there are limits to science. "Even if there is only one possible unified theory, it is just a set of rules and equations. What is it that breathes fire into the equations and makes a universe for them to describe?" Or from his hugely popular but rarely read book *A Brief History of Time* (a running joke Hawking found humorous): "It would be very difficult to explain why the universe should have begun in just this way, except as the act of a God who intended to create beings like us."[4] So much for science explaining all, once we get to it.

A compelling counter to scientific materialism exists in our empirical awareness of the anthropic components.[5] The anthropic components are basically the many states of astonishing equilibrium that exist throughout the universe and on earth for no particular reason except perhaps to make life possible—that is, human-centric creature that I am, our life, your life, as exists at every moment from the big bang up to and including this precise moment you read and breathe and curse me. To say we are *unlikely* to have come into being, to have developed singularly into human beings, and to miraculously continue to thrive as we do is the scientific understatement of all time. And to avoid acknowledging Hawking's most fundamental scientific question of all time, to build scientific theories on foundations of avoidance is to create a metaphoric house of straw. Scientific truth ain't of our choosing any more than is the existence or non-existence of God.

Anthropic components are sometimes referred as the Goldilocks effect—the earth is not too hot and not too cold—but are actually far more dramatic and frankly impossible, as odds go. Each of the numerous components must be precisely as they are, or life cannot exist—for example, earth's distance from the sun for precise temperature, the moon's distance from earth for precision of ocean tides and gravitational functioning. Remember, each individual component is spectacularly unlikely if one is talking the language of chance, and it must be emphasized that life only exists because **all** unlikely components work, and we need all of them in order to live. The scientific truth of our existence on earth is that it is impossible if not for the scientific fact that we exist on earth. It seems that scientific truth as exists, which may be apart from scientific thinking as practised, requires the acceptance of contradiction.

Professor Dawkins repeatedly chastises those whose consciousness have not risen in recognition of the power of natural selection to flatten the improbability of life's extraordinary diversity on earth. And, of course, he makes a strong point based on science. But what is far more difficult to account for, what remains inexplicable, is the fact that life ever began. And what kind of odds were the advent of life with anthropic

---

4. Stephen Hawking, *A Brief History of Time* (New York: Bantam Books, 1998), 144.
5. See Hugh Ross, *The Creator and the Cosmos: How the Greatest Scientific Discoveries of the Century Reveal God* (Colorado Springs: NavPress Publishing, 1993), for a fulsome explanation of anthropic components' staggering complexity and harmony.

components sustaining the infinitesimally thin margins that constitute conditions for existence? Two to one? One hundred to one? Why do Dawkins, Kraus, and all skirt the issue of how bloody unlikely, left to chance, the fact of our life is, inventing multiverses along with other non-empirical fantastical theories that serve to titillate and confound but not engage?

In *Darwin Devolves*, biologist Michael Behe cites bioinformatician Eugene Koonin as working out the probability of life arising on its own to be 10 to the 1,018rd power.[6] If even remotely predictive, this figure indicates that life's humble beginnings faced greater odds than picking a single designated grain of sand from all the sand in the world. Or to borrow from an oft used concept attributed to physicist Fred Hoyle: life on earth was less likely to just spring into existence than for a tornado to pass through a junkyard and assemble a Boeing 747. We haven't just beat the odds; humans have won a trillion trillion trillion lotteries in a row with no end in sight, and yet Dawkins explains anthropic components and the beginning of life on earth as simply scientific stuff that happens and which we will fully understand once science gets to it. It is a "gap" to be filled in, in time. *Oh yeah*, he concedes, *I guess we're a wee bit lucky*.

So, in a funny kind of way, speculation on the arbitrary and infinite multiverse, and really any other theory, makes sense. Only wild speculation allows you, I, respected scientists, to dodge impossible odds and make their case within the confines of scientific materialism. And yet, Koonin's odds would be just about the same as those used by atheists to allow for the existence of God. The only difference is that the anthropic components are science, whereas an uncompromising dismissal of God is actually antithetical to science. What is known in science with application of logic speaks to the existence of God, same for what is unknown. That is, unknown is not simply what science will solve in time; unknown may be what science cannot solve because it is unknowable. Science will never solve how anthropic components came together to work as they do and, importantly, in harmony, to sustain our astonishingly precarious existence. *But for the grace of God* is our every-second reality to be aware of, to wonder at, not to solve. But that should not keep us from trying. And once all the trying has been reflected upon, we need conclusions to be dispassionate and empirical rather than dismissive and ideological.

One day I was working a whirlwind shift, no break, no time to think about no break, and I thought, *Chris is gone*. I was informed that he had been gone for two weeks. We were assigned to different people each shift, unlike the nursing staff, whose patients tended to be the same for their rehab duration. I vaguely thought that since I had not been assigned to Chris, it was no wonder I hadn't noticed he was gone. But no, the truth is, I had not thought about Chris, because I had just not thought about Chris. He left rehab as soon as he could talk or communicate through

6. Michael J. Behe, *Darwin Devolves: The New Science About DNA That Challenges Evolution* (New York: HarperOne, 2019), 105.

heavy silence that he wanted out. I never saw him again and have no idea what became of his life. We were not friends; there is no reason I would know anything.

Still, these decades later, I wonder what happened to Chris, even if it took me two weeks to notice that he, who lived, breathed, and struggled right under my nose, was gone. What does it mean when people imperceptibly cruise into our consciousness, leave deep footprints, and then vacate without a trace? But of course, there is always a trace. The recording and meaning of what we do and don't do began long before the digital assignment, and continues to this day. Meaning is not uncompacting s**t; it exists in doing what must be done for whomever God places in our path, and the responsibility for that encounter never fully ends. It is the good news for spiritual subversives and an inconvenient truth for moderns, to be avoided or expunged from the record. Still, if we are what we do and not what we accumulate, the record exists.

• • •

I had found useful work, and although I completed two graduate degrees, real was so much more compelling than theory. It may be that wanting to find useful work comes from deep-seated feelings of being useless. Which of course we are until we do something useful. A healthy dose of low self-esteem helps. The self-esteem industry thinks that the worst thing that can happen to a young person is to have low self-esteem, and I think that the worst thing that can happen to a young person is to have high self-esteem. The cure for low self-esteem is to do something useful; there is no cure for high self-esteem. (Yes, I'm being mildly facetious in aspiring to C. S. Lewis: "True humility is not thinking less of yourself; it is thinking of yourself less.")

But there was something else. I was drawn to this work because of family. My dad died the month I became an orderly. In 1939, when he was 18, he had enlisted in the navy, as was the thing to do in 1939, as is not understood much anymore because all war is now naively believed to be wrong. On a ship in the navy, Dad loved a storm at sea. Seems innocent enough, but the Dad we knew didn't indulge such passions, approached all situations with utilitarian caution. He had a reason most of the time for not doing whatever was being proposed. Everything had to make sense, which for a kid doesn't allow for much. The key for us growing up was to not ask for permission.

For a teenager to go into the navy during wartime could not have been easy, but it must have made sense, even before everything had to make sense. Dad's family was poor, the thirties had been a depressed decade, life was hard, opportunity was non-existent. Dad had a camera and photographed and neatly chronicled his navy convoy travels across the Atlantic in 1939 and 1940. The photos capture a young man in his element, thriving with adventure, useful occupation, and three square meals a day, something never assured in his pre-war circumstances. One night he goes out in a storm and is thrown against a guardrail and breaks his back, and his life, as he knew it, is over.

35

Dad had crushed several vertebrae and was operated on by the world-renowned neurosurgeon Dr. Wilder Penfield, followed by a year of rehab at the Montreal Neurological Institute. Dad had several spinal fusions, forgoing the last surgery, which was considered too risky and could quite possibility have left him a paraplegic. Dad's accident and surgeries made him a celebrity of sorts in an impersonal way, as his case was featured in medical textbooks of the day. Dad's surgeries left him very little ability to turn his back or neck and a lifelong problem with pain. Still, he could walk, and as soon as possible he went back to active duty, training fellow seamen as a flagman. It was the trifecta of broken back, emphysema, and self-medicating for pain that caused Dad's early death in 1980, at age 59.

But of course, one doesn't simply die 40 years after an accident. There is that detail about living until we get to death. The short version is, he suffered. Watching Dad wasting away and struggling to breathe made an impression. I remember when I was about 10 feeling a deep catch in my throat, not a sore throat but a strain that made it hard to breathe. Mom listened, concerned; Dad swatted down the ridiculous notion, and the notion went away, or at least went somewhere. Dad was right that I didn't need a doctor; I needed to dispel the image of Dad sitting in a chair, a portrait of exertion, drawing rapid, shallow, and painful breaths from one moment to the next.

Still, I could not unsee the image, and the same remains true today. It would not have been right for me to have not seen Dad as he was, just as it would not be right for me to have forgotten. In his unemotive way, Dad's shallow breath was his deepest articulation. It only occurred to me in writing this account that my breathing episode was a psychosomatic response to Dad's condition—that thing before us that no one talked about, including during the month of August 1980, as he lay dying in hospital, where I visited him when I wasn't working at the other hospital I now worked at as an orderly. Obvious today. It seems we see least often what is right before our eyes.

In addition to my new job and Dad's decline, I took on something else to complete my own trifecta. That same month I began a distance running career, competing for 30 years; it's still a daily habit, but now as a non-competitive activity with my dog, Zigo. So yes, meeting Chris afforded an opportunity to be useful, but it was more than that. In Dad's final month of limited mobility and in my first month witnessing complete immobility, I found a way to emote, equal parts exercise and exorcise, my deepest fear. Courageous Chris—they were all spectacularly courageous—scared me for what common experience could inflict upon a decent person; immobility scared me, which for someone who cannot sit still must be particularly acute; and Dad's death scared me for what pain and suffering come to. It just seemed then to end. So, I ran, and ran away.

But mobilizing against immobility doesn't really work. We talk about walking a mile in someone else's shoes, but our feet rarely fit their shoes. We can't live someone else's life, it is true, but part of the distance that exists between human beings is due to our unwillingness to extend ourselves to bridge the gap. That is our contradiction—desire and resistance, empathy and fear at odds, for most of our lives. Superficially, we deny this, but at a deeper level we intuit its truth, and at the deepest level we know that only a few will find a way to fully connect and articulate. Still, for all the separateness in life, there is hope. The world can turn on a singular distilled act of compassion. Perhaps most important while we work on compassion is this: *always search for the person beneath the circumstances.*

Terry was as likeable a guy as they come. Tough to be, for most; almost impossible for a young man who wakes up to profound loss of his own making (at least that is the conventional view, though another explanation of the non-material world may lurk deeper). Terry's accident was not as a result of drinking, the common assumed cause for a single car accident late at night. No, Terry fell asleep at the wheel, for the third time, third time very unlucky—another unfortunate trifecta. He could joke about this, and really anything else about his life as a patient on the ward. For all the seriousness of his situation, he didn't take himself too seriously. Frivolous humour does not predict depth of feeling.

Humour, as applied to self-deprecation, is a great defence against life's vicissitudes. But at some point, it is hard not to wake up to the cards one has been dealt. The rehab process is long for traumatic spinal cord injury, measured in months not weeks. Immobility, invasive daily rituals, involuntary shared quarters, and the endless distraction of therapies conspire to make life on the ward suffocating and narrow. For all the best efforts from staff, the route to independence is tortuously long. Finally, having achieved some stability, and with the requisite support in place, it is time for the first weekend home. This is an event that is faced with some trepidation and great expectations.

There are logistical considerations such as getting into the house or apartment, the ability to negotiate bathroom and kitchen where accessibility is likely most challenging, medications to dispense, bowel and bladder issues to manage, etc. Often accessibility is very problematic such a short time after injury, but for that first visit, friends and family usually rally, in large numbers, and obstacles are dealt with. There is no permanent solution in having one's personal army carry the spinal cord injured person up stairs that one used to take two or three at a time. It is nice that people respond, especially after months of being sympathetic but useless on the sidelines. It is heartwarming, but the best of—and we are talking genuine love— weekend staging intentions cannot translate into how the injured person is able to build a new life.

Everyone is well-meaning, wanting to contribute, wanting to create some semblance of what life was like before, if only for that first weekend home. But the centre will not hold. Exuberance is not enough, and sometimes it is too much. Terry, from a small town outside of Ottawa, had a crew of brothers and many friends to help with any and all barriers. Most important, everyone would be together again, just like it used to be.

Terry had fantasized on the ward about music, home cooking, and beer because none were available there, and the ward was not home. But as Terry's car drove down familiar streets to his house, as he crossed the threshold into his house, courtesy of physical exertion from exuberant brothers, as he looked out from the living room window into the yard where he and his brothers roughhoused their way through life, he had feelings. Going home is very emotional, but Terry was not used to having uncomfortable feelings, especially about his home and family. The accident, the rehab gig, had been tough, but he and his family had sucked it up their whole lives, and this was supposed to be an extension of the same.

Terry grinned and laughed and talked. He ate home-cooked food and drank beer, encouraged by everyone to catch up with the essentials of life denied in hospital. The homecoming was a success, except that somehow home was not home, and now Terry knew it never would be again. Still, Terry did not tell anyone what he felt and had no intention of telling a therapist at the rehab centre when he got back. The next day and night featured more people and more catching up with people. This was Terry's homecoming, and people had always been drawn to him.

I was working the Sunday evening shift when Terry came back to the ward after his first weekend home. He arrived back at the expected time, around 8 p.m. Terry was assigned to me. He was always easy to get along with. But the look on his face as he came off the elevator was not easy.

It had started during the drive home. Too much food and beer, too little schedule, hard to know. It was horribly unfair for his first weekend home, first time being reacquainted with a thin version of normalcy in many months. It was what it was, and it was obvious without Terry saying a word, not talking likely being his only relief of the evening. Terry had s**t himself, diarrhea technically, from head to toe. No sensation while doing it, no way to prevent it, and no way to hide the smell once it spread its foul wings. It had been a long car ride.

Without a word we went into his room, which mercifully was empty of the three other occupants. Twenty minutes later Terry was verging on feeling human again, but he was far from being his easygoing self. Something had changed on that first weekend home. There was a deep demarcation between his old life and the one he now faced. Diarrhea punctuated that fact, but it was not the fact. His family understood as well. They were salt of the earth, willing to do anything for their son and brother. The party was over, and they could not help him. From the corridor, as family members prepared to leave, empty words were punctuated by filler grunts and polite echoey coughs. The inarticulate speech of the heart has these guttural glimpses, poignant and raw.

Orderlies are good at doing casual. No big deal, I say, it's what we do, I was bored anyway. Terry knows I bulls**t, but at least awkward is over. He is staying in bed. It's been an exhausting weekend, and he has this disorienting feeling of hating this place yet sensing he cannot be elsewhere. He tries to push this thought away, and the phone rings. It is his girlfriend. His high school sweetheart, who did not go away to school as planned because of his accident in June. He had told her to go, but she had hunkered down and refused to go then, even though there was no guarantee that her spot in the prestigious physiotherapy program could be deferred. The program had very exacting standards, with very limited enrolment, and ironically it was training for the therapy that Terry was going to need most often in life. Generally, requests for deferment were turned down, but a compromise had been offered.

Terry assured her that she should take the offer; she resisted, but they both knew she had to take it, and they both knew that it was the end of their relationship. She needed his permission; he could not withhold it. Some people can only do the right thing, regardless of personal cost.

Orderlies were also good at creeping just outside the perimeter, there if needed, non-existent if not. Terry cried. Most men don't cry easily, and because of that, the act of crying can be acutely painful. Terry cried as never before, and not in a cathartic way. He had hit bottom. As the saying goes, there is nowhere else to go but up. As I left my shift that night I wasn't so sure hitting bottom necessitated coming back up. But I always had the luxury, indulgence, call it what you will, of vacating strife for life, and as always, the first breath of cool night air hit me like a cannon of relief, guilt, a proverbial slap in the grateful face. These years later the image of gentle, likeable Terry crushed by brutal facts of life in the material world burns.

Terry was back to being easy the next shift I worked with him. Easy to work with, easy manner, big smile. Same for every time I saw him after his rehab days for the next almost 25 years, until he died suddenly at age 43. He had been young when injured, like so many others, and had watched his life from the sidelines until it just ended. It was unexpected and no surprise.

We are witnessing the first generation of high-level quadriplegics who are living significantly beyond the time of their traumatic accident. Though Dr. Penfield's surgeries at the Montreal Neurological Institute were innovative in the 1940s, spinal fusion was relatively primitive. Stabilizing the spinal column for high-level quadriplegics is more challenging than spinal fusion, even before getting to the ongoing issues of kidney and liver function and management of skin and muscle problems that come from too little movement and too much sitting in one place for too long.

Given how bloody difficult the whole ball of wax is, it is astonishing how many people live reasonably long and productive lives. Quadriplegics wake in hospital one day, say age 18, after driving under the influence of alcohol or drugs on high school graduation night, or diving into shallow water, or more recently an accident from a multiplicity of technological distractions, or none of the above but simply an inexplicable moment of inattention, and in waking are attached to a body whose immobility is antithetical to every instinct and habit of their young lives. Not my assessment but what is communicated from the silent scream heard on the ward in the early weeks. Still, quadriplegics learn the impossible—and in pulling off the impossible, it cannot be said often enough, *they go out and do it again every hour of every day*.

Many have carried off the miracle 30 or 40 years beyond the age of innocence, and counting. Still, some can't bring themselves to manage and care enough to maximize longevity. Bed sores, kidney problems, too much drinking, not enough fluids. Management is important, I guess, but for some management isn't life. With a life sentence of treading water, for some it's easier to simply allow oneself to be gently pulled under, and who can blame them? For those who fight, decades on, setting records for longevity, reconciling deeply feeling mind to unfeeling body, you can't help thinking, what bloody admirable toughness, guts, and personal integrity it must take. There is mystery in this, the *this* being more, not less, mysterious for its appearance of common. It happens commonly but is not common.

Dad's post-accident forty-year ordeal aged him. He looked 80 and moved like he was 100. At his funeral, a couple of old friends drifted in, no idea who they were, not sure they said. They would have been about his age, and it occurred to me that Dad could have been like them, upright, still a going concern, not spent. Each had something to say about Dad back before the war when they were teenagers together. They hadn't known Dad later in life and were disconnected from all we knew of him. Apparently, Dad had been a great athlete—gymnastics, hockey, or anything in the park and in the "hood." He'd been good or best at whatever he turned his mind or body to. He loved a game, and he loved to move. The dad we knew always took his car to get cigarettes at the corner store one block away and disparaged exercise without utilitarian purpose.

The young guys on the spinal cord unit never knew who they might have become. I suppose that is true for all of us. We all have a sense of the *other*, if only we'd made different choices, had better luck. But for those who lose everything they have ever valued or have been able to define themselves by, the loss is particularly acute, the spectra of *other* lingering, returning, or haunting throughout the years. Even for those who extract a life from the embers of circumstance against achingly difficult odds and achieve a higher version of themselves than ever would have been possible without adversity, it is difficult not to equate self with loss. My quadriplegic friends are not different than any of us, ultimately; they just live life distilled to the elemental core. We are not simply the losses that happened to us; we are how we played the cards we were dealt. Character.

Watching Dad from earliest memory until his death when I was 25 had an effect, though to this day I'm not exactly sure what it was. Dad's was a stony inarticulate silence, which I wish I'd been able to penetrate. I wish I'd been able to help. I didn't kid myself about being able to help those early spinal cord patients, though at least on the ward I wasn't still and wasn't silent. No real help, but not useless—a compromise I clung to.

On a spinal cord ward, you don't meet paralysis and immobility. You meet doers, athletes, risk takers, people who loved movement and took life by the horns. And the separation and assumptions that flow into the wake of traumatic spinal cord injury have to be resisted for the duration. Medical staff and therapists tend to urge "the patient" to embrace the new reality of self, in order to best get on with the life that remains. I'm not so sure. I'm not sure that the former self has to be abandoned, is ever over. I would have liked to know more about who the young quads were who were patients before they knew what a patient was. It might be healthy to occasionally allow in the entire person—present circumstances along with the *other* from another time—who is more than just a ghost to be chased away by the light of dawn. In time, everything will be utterly transformed, and for all the emphasis on being in the moment, it is not enough. We are our long-ragged memory; our narrative is a full book, each past or future chapter as important as the one we find ourselves in.

In the first five minutes of my first shift as Chris endured the indignity of a stranger performing the necessary ritual in the transformed life that was to be his, he might have wanted to escape mindfulness. But to what? Where would his mind go? Did it matter what happened to him, or was it just something to endure until oblivion? It is of course a question of meaning. Perhaps the existential question is this: Was Chris a physically wounded person who was about to be tested to the limit, for whom courage would be required every hour of every day in a way few of us would ever see, could ever imagine, and whose experience even he would be at a loss to articulate from the depth of an intact, soaring soul; or was he no more than the offensive fecal matter pulled from his a*s, to be dumped and redistributed back into the universe where energy is neither created nor lost, where you are neither loved not hated, where life and death are just cells that were and are no more, the interchange between swirling atoms just part of the indifferent, non-judgmental universe, all things being equal, essence being essentially non-existent? The simple answer to this long-winded question we are all tasked to answer is the purpose of our life, is why Chris ultimately is on our collective path, is why he matters.

Chapter Two

"NO BIG DEAL"

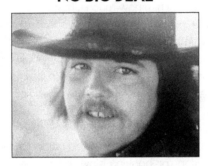

"Real friendship or love is not manufactured or achieved by an
act of will or intention. Friendship is always an act of recognition."
John O'Donohue, Irish writer, philosopher, Christian mystic (1956–2008)

I have a clear memory of Paul. He is sitting alone, waiting for me in his wheelchair at the dreaded twenty-mile mark and lowest point on the course. Same for where my mind was in the race before the ascent at Parliament Hill. Twenty miles is a long way to have run hard, both psychologically and physically. The conventional wisdom is, at 20 miles into a marathon the second and hardest half of the race begins.

There were many thousands of people running in the marathon, mostly in big and small groups, together according to ability. I somehow always managed to get caught alone, strung out a couple hundred metres from the leaders, usually finishing in the top ten but never leading or running with any other lonely stranger. I suffered alone.

Twenty-six miles or forty-two kilometres watching someone's struggling a*s, as the guy behind me watches mine. You'd think one or the other would slow down or speed up to get company, but no. Long-distance running is not only lonely; running alone at 20 miles is the equivalent of dropping in the desert and watching buzzards circling overhead.

While I always said, "Doesn't matter," "Don't come out," and "Don't need a cheer," I wasn't exactly being honest. A heartfelt cheer at a low point helps galvanize body and mind, both wanting to capitulate to entropy creep and call it quits. Some parts of the course were crowded with cheering people, but at other parts, and notably at the twenty-mile mark, there were too few people and still too much distance. There was no maddening crowd, which was maddening. Paul knew this, and his lonely vigilance for nothing more than a lonelier quick glance sideways gave me the strength to resist quitting, to finish. Seems a small thing, him coming out then and to that spot, but no, when you are about to break, not unlike while interrogated under torture, you will grasp at anything to get from this one moment to the next. The thought *I'll never do this again* is no insulation against present-moment self-inflicted suffering.

I don't remember what Paul actually said to me in flight; couldn't have been much. I don't remember telling him how much it meant to me. I should have told him how much it meant to me. He didn't need encouragement or validation to show up; he just showed up every time. "No big deal," he'd say, though I think Woodie Allen is credited with saying, "Eighty percent of success is just showing up." Even if showing up is not a big deal—though it is—not showing up in life is.

What was a big deal was planning to get to that spot on the course at that precise moment. These casual appearances required booking an attendant at least three hours earlier than on a normal Sunday morning, getting dressing, conducting bowel and bladder routines, arranging transportation to the exact place, in his adapted van when working, or booking slow, often late, inconsistent accessible public transportation when not, and finding a disabled parking spot with an extra wide space for electric wheelchair egress while hoping that some schmuck hadn't stolen it on the assumption that people in wheelchairs don't come to running events. And then there were the contingencies of weather, with both rain and heat being a problem, and always the heavy aggravation if keys are dropped or if there is a urine leak—there really are too many possibilities to come up with a plan for all. Paul had to plan for everything and then resolve to put up with whatever other new ravages to his person presented themselves, as they often did, spontaneity being 15 years in the past. Determined not to be late, he had to sit and wait—estimated time of arrival being difficult to predict—for hours in order to give seconds of support. How could he not know I cared?

For all that, he knew my running pedigree; that is, he knew what pace I would be running, expected time of arrival if the race started on time, what times I had run in previous races, my PBs (personal bests) for all distances, and especially what I hoped to accomplish that day if the stars aligned, which I wouldn't admit to anyone else for fear of jinxing my race. He knew my training times, steady runs, track times, and cross country repeat loops in the arboretum. He asked lots of questions, was genuinely interested in something that is not very interesting, and once answered, it was in the vault for later perfect recall.

That last marathon was bad. I'd gone out hard, determined to stay with the leaders, determined to reach the unstated goal of breaking two hours, twenty minutes, but I used too much energy too early on, unwise in distance races, a recipe for disaster in a marathon. Before the half-marathon mark, I was finished, but Irish Catholic perversity in full flight, I gutted out the second half, fading badly, finishing on a day it would have been wise to quit. I was maybe fifth or sixth place, time of 2:24 for the second time in three years, the hoped for breakthrough not happening, with collapse into the arms of a volunteer as expected from everyone who watched me in the previous three marathon finishes. Through the haze of exhaustion, I heard, without seeing, a medical tent volunteer say, "Oh yeah, he does that every year; take him to the tent," which motivated me to stand somewhat straight and wobble in the opposite direction.

While clinging to the notion of breakthrough, I'd always prided myself on getting decent results on low mileage. I averaged a focused 80 kilometres each week during my competitive days, which was enough for racing 10Ks and even half-marathons, but the marathon is another beast altogether. Marathon winners tend to do at least 160 kilometres a week, some far more. Even doing the odd continuous 40 kilometre training run did not make up for the fact that the marathon is not satisfied by quality alone and demands a healthy chunk of quantity to make one competitive.

I wanted to believe I could compete on a diet of 80 kilometres because that is all I could handle alongside a full-time job and two young children. Paul and I talked about *the problem,* and he had several insightful suggestions, which coming from him I considered carefully. His suggestions had to do with making structural changes, but in the end, I realized that it was not a structural problem; it was not even a problem. I really didn't want to run any more than 80 kilometres a week, and whenever I tended towards higher mileage, my immune system would let me know it was not pleased. The obvious answer came a year or two later: quit the marathon and compete at what was working, which were all the other, shorter and yet significantly long, distances.

Once I made that decision—25 kilometres into a 35-kilometre training run, along the canal in Ottawa at the big curve on Queen Elizabeth Drive, in front of a wooden park bench—I was fine. I never ran the marathon again, never missed it, and had personal best times for every other distance I competed in that year. Still, thoughts of the marathon leave me guilty to this day.

The previous August I had been training for the Montreal marathon and had to get my longest run in before tapering—that is, before lowering the length of my runs down as the race got closer in order to be both fit and rested. My final 40-kilometre training run was scheduled for a late Saturday in August, a scorcher, and coincidentally Paul's wedding day.

Paul, good-looking, witty, a willing listener, and charming to both girls and guys, had met and was about to marry a babe who was also a teacher and nice person. This was no sympathy relationship. Women loved this guy. I should not have run a torturous 40 kilometre run in hot conditions on Paul's wedding day. I should have planned for his wedding as much as Paul had planned for my marathon. No, that doesn't make sense. His planning was formidable; all I had to do was not run so long. That should not have been difficult.

But I did the long run, and throughout the afternoon into evening I realized I had induced a fever. There was a babysitting issue too, which was not a reason but with two daughters sufficed as not one but two excuses. I didn't drink enough water that day, often weighing in at a full five pounds less post-run than pre-run. We had been rushed getting to the wedding because the run took two and a half hours and I had not gotten up in time to get it done early—which also meant I ran when the temperature was highest, which exacerbated my pathetic unnecessary feverish symptoms.

I didn't prepare for Paul's wedding; I gutted my way through it, which had been my modus operandi my whole life. Why enjoy life when you can suffer? Shortly after dinner, early into the reception, we made our excuses and left. We had a couple of kids to get back to, after all. It sounded like a poor excuse then, and nothing has changed in over 30 years, including forgiving myself. Not that there was anything to forgive from Paul's point of view. But on this occasion, he was wrong. The training didn't matter; the wedding did. Attending and celebrating in life are not the same thing.

And this was *Paul's* wedding. I should have seen this as the eighth wonder of the world. Not because a quadriplegic found a nice girl to marry him. No, the wonder of it was that he was able to pull his life back into a degree of normalcy after enduring the inexplicable. The inexplicable happened in the form of an astonishingly rare aneurysm in his neck, which was discovered when he was 19 years old, that ruptured two years later, leaving him a high-level quadriplegic. This isn't supposed to happen to young athletic people. How does anyone cope?

Paul had extraordinary family support, which is essential, but the years 19 to 21 are exactly when the universe is titling towards freedom and independence, basically when young cocky guys tell the world just how infallible they are. The infallibility shtick is an illusion, but the young guy is supposed to have some time to unravel cockiness, to have fun before moving from hubris to humility.

The best families in the world—and Paul had the best—don't wait by the proverbial bedside as passive bystanders. Still, doing everything that can be done cannot undo what has been done. Which gets to the core of Paul, the people in this book, and my fascination with all the miraculous humans I have met and worked with for the last 30 years. I don't understand what the mystery is, just that there is one. Paul's solitary view from the deep impenetrable place in which he lived and his ability to perceive it as otherwise took character infused with—what? The secular view puts it into psychological terms, resiliency and courage certainly. But there has to be something more, perhaps grace. Grace is not outside of self, is not someone else doing the job, the one that the person is incapable of doing. Grace is given; it is rare; it is not earned so much as reflective of character, the striving for one's higher self; and decades later it continues to send out concentric waves that the inarticulate speech of my still stubborn heart strains to hear and can never ignore.

I liked him the moment we met, admired him in the years that followed, but only came to see the width and breadth of Paul long after he had died. While finishing grad school and working as an orderly, I answered a call for volunteers from a sign he'd put up in the university. Paul was coordinator for the disabled but no longer needed volunteers since he was days away from moving on to another job. But if not for that impulse to volunteer, my life would have been much different. After our first meeting we agreed to keep in touch, and Paul asked if he could recommend me for the job he was vacating. I agreed and even managed to do his old job half-time while continuing as an orderly and grad student. The coordination half-time job went from 9 a.m. until 1 p.m., evening orderly shifts were 3 p.m. until 11 p.m., and class attendance was non-existent. How was that even possible, I have been challenged. Not over-thinking helped. Also grades for the four graduate courses I was enrolled in were 100 percent based on writing research papers, which, if nothing else, I had learned to do quickly. Throw in marathon training, and you could say I was busy, though I didn't think much of it at the time. Whether Paul didn't think about it too much or had far-reaching insight, he had launched my career.

Every week after that, without fail, Paul and I talked during work, about work. He always opening up conversation with the words "How goes the battle?" And whatever else life is, it is a battle—not to disparage, take for granted, or complain about—but all of the good, the bad, and the ugly was somehow made more endurable or illuminated by articulating battle lines, strategies, plans of attack, and defensive positions. We were both new in our jobs, for which there was no manual or established standards of practice. We asked each how the other might handle an anticipated situation, and we adjusted our thinking based on input received. Add to the conversation home life, future plans, and aspirations, commonalities and differences all part of free-flowing, comfortable, and intense never-ending discussion. I miss the world of conversation.

Which is why I was surprised during this time when someone asked a question about our friendship: Does Paul, immobile as he is, live vicariously through you as a mobile runner? I don't remember who asked, but I do remember I didn't respond well. It was a dumb-a**ed question that illustrated the unnecessary distance that can come into any relationship because of perceived difference. Paul was interested in me and probably wanted to make sure the issue of mobility didn't cause distance— he never said so, but I suspect he'd had too much of that. I never said so, but I didn't want the issue of immobility to cause distance either, so between common values and true comfort with each other, our friendship grew. We are not simply a culmination of the cards we have been dealt; balance in any relationship is not determined by our worldly circumstances.

In counselling psychology, that sweet spot optimal for best outcomes is dependent upon the establishment of a therapeutic alliance. That alliance is primarily a one-way benefit from therapist to client. Occasionally—and yes, shockingly even between guys—it is possible to create a two-way therapeutic alliance—that is, real friendship, support, and deep mutual understanding without misunderstanding, unaltered by outside people, events, or—persistent problem especially for guys—competition, come h**l or high water, which guys prefer to say over unconditional love. Still, Paul and I had the *that* of which that is.

Mostly because of Paul. We were both from that Irish Catholic emotionally retentive background, but while I was stereotypical of my stock, he was the spectacular exception. He did *intimate*, that guy-style rarity; I meekly followed, which was easy because it was hard not to respond to Paul. We all respond well to people who instinctively pull us out of our lower, more fearful selves. We just don't meet people who can do that very often. Paul was capable of being that other Irish Catholic type, warm, talkative, with a touch of Irish blarney. This without an ounce of insincerity, just part of the charm.

It is no exaggeration to say that in those early years, Paul prevented me from bailing from working in the disability arena. An aspect of the disability movement emerging in 1980s was an expectation that people working in the field of disability have a disability. I felt the pressure of being a TABB (a term coined by my first student, Dennis, meaning Temporarily Able-Bodied B*****d). I loved the work, which had a very real pioneering element to it, but I felt like a fraud. Paul would have none of it. He said it was the work that you do and not who you are that matters. He reminded me that if he was not simply the product of his various parts, chances, and circumstances, neither was I. I always felt better after talking to Paul, felt like plunging back into battle. Paul would not allow me the indulgence of slinking away from what he considered an identity politics problem, decades before the term was coined. He had no tolerance for divisive identity obsession, insisting that any movement with value is actually an alliance of people from all walks of life, including those not walking. I have always been grateful to Paul for that, that being permission to continue to work without being consumed by guilt.

Still, more guilt lingers. I know that in the nihilistic modern world in which we dwell, we are supposed to have expunged guilt as a useless emotion. Life is about self-actualization and experience in the mindful now. What has passed has passed. Blame, and especially self-blame, is for suckers. I am so square and archaic that I believe guilt can be important, not to wallow in but to acknowledge and learn from. We humans have the potential to be liberated or imprisoned by conscience; liberation is awareness; imprisonment is the inability to acknowledge or articulate what we become aware of.

I am thinking and writing these too-serious thoughts while sitting in a café at a resort in Cuba, on a perfect March morning, after running barefoot along that sweet spot where ocean waters recede, exposing hard packed cool sand. Back home, it is minus 30, before factoring in wind chill; here I never bother to check, since days flow from one to the other with little variation to pleasing temperature and sunny skies. People who come here have no past. The holiday all-inclusive world excludes all that is not happening during their hard-earned week of indulgence. We need to forget sometimes. We need to move on from bad things that happened. But the actual application of mindfulness/mindlessness can lead to amnesia about who we are. The trajectory of our lives includes that we lose everything—a terrible thought during an all-inclusive holiday—including the chance to say what needs to be said, which is central to life's purpose and, not coincidently, this book.

Saying what needs to be said is one of the most difficult tasks in life, right up until we lose someone we didn't say what needed to be said to, at which precise moment it is the easiest and most compelling action we didn't take. How's that for irony? The only way I can work out some of the things I've done or haven't done in life is to feel guilty afterwards, even long after the fact. Such is the perversity of my thinking. In the mindlessness of an all-inclusive I could not get past the past, as I never can, and I thought about Paul, 30 years tumbling backwards with eerie precision. I was not much of an all-inclusive conversationalist.

On one afternoon of eerie precision, Paul called me at work. He did not ask "How goes the battle?" which should have been an obvious clue. He asked if I could meet him at his house. I agreed without asking why he was not at work that day. I set out immediately but needed gas and stopped at a station that included a free car wash with every fill up. I decided to take the car wash, likely only one of two washes my old Toyota 4 Runner ever had. To this day I'm not clear in my own mind why I took the car wash.

I arrived at Paul's house, only a couple houses removed from his parents' house where he had grown up. He waited inside framed by the large picture window of his living room. For almost an hour he had been marinating in his own urine. I entered the room and noticed his dripping pants, as he looked outside at my still dripping truck. Six self-incriminating words cut into my chest from Paul's innocuous question: "You stopped for a car wash?" I hear the words still.

Obviously, Paul's catheter had either broken or fallen off, and whatever Paul's reason for being home, his attendant was not scheduled to return again until evening. Paul had called me because he was stranded. Everything Paul was able to still do in life was compromised. Spontaneity was almost non-existent; all of life's functions had to be planned, with little or no room for error. This formidable aggravation prevents many people with high-level physical disabilities from pursuing adventure and travel. For most, just getting through the day is an adventure in advanced aggravation. It is antithetical to the all-inclusive.

And then there is the heightened risk to just about every aspect of movement and travel. Still, Paul was a risk-taker and adventurer, and most of all, he wanted to be where his people were.

His people constituted a wide circle of humanity. His infamous charm to which I have alluded was fundamentally based on the comfort he was able to project about himself to others, all others. People were drawn to him, saw him even when it would have been easier to look through him, as so many of us do to people who unknowingly represent our deep-seated fears.

Paul's two brothers never stopped seeing him. One summer just after Paul became a quadriplegic, his older brother, Donald, and younger, Jerome, decided that the three Menton boys needed a raucous road trip. This was 1976, before vans or much of anything was accessible. Still, challenging road trips were what young guys did before the word *travel* was contaminated by the passive and seductive aforementioned all-inclusive.

Paul's mother was furious. The care of a quadriplegic, especially then, was precarious at best, mostly downright risky, requiring constant vigilance, even in a medical facility. Paul was among the first generation of spinal cord injured, primarily young men, who did not die shortly after injury. The question of life expectancy was unknown to doctors, medical staff, patients, and families. Medical interventions had been revolutionized since the Second World War: surgery to stabilize the spinal column; care of bowel, bladder, kidneys, and skin; rehabilitation techniques; and drugs to limit infection, control spasms, assist with organ function, and treat depression. Outside of hospital and rehabilitation facilities, the world was totally unprepared for these young accessibility pioneers, just as they were unprepared to be pioneers, had no idea they were pioneers.

The brothers understood much and expressed little. Words could not express; sometimes inarticulate speech is best expressed in action. As long as Paul was alive—and that was a miracle in itself—they had to find a kernel of normalcy within this horror that had descended upon them. The road trip was not pretend, was not going to be a patronizing version of what they understood a road trip to be, and they were determined, Paul most of all, to take six weeks and go from eastern Ontario to the far west, ending at the Pacific Ocean, I guess the reasoning being that travelling less than a five-figure number of kilometres is not a road trip but just a Sunday drive. Normalcy required extremity. Paul's new condition was not going to change the definition of *road trip*, vintage 1970s.

Paul's dad, Joe, came around once confronted with Paul's determination, but Paul's mother, Phyllis, could not become reconciled to the madness that had descended upon her boys. And it was madness; equally so, it needed to be done. Paul, trying to cope with his new life, and his brothers, who felt useless to help Paul cope with his new life, needed to do something. At the same time, Paul's mother could not be faulted for thinking the plan may have had some deficiencies. The three brothers were going to travel in a van that had faulty brakes that they did not intend to fully fix because they couldn't afford the actual needed repair. Joe and his boys spent an inordinate amount of time tinkering with the brakes before the departure but never could quite figure out the problem. So rather than sweat the small stuff, the Menton brothers developed a method of pumping the brakes into submission, which made for particularly interesting driving as they descended from the Rockies.

It should be mentioned that deficient as their plan may have seemed, and decrepit as their Volkswagen van was, the three Menton brothers made it all the way to the Pacific Ocean and, to their mother's everlasting relief, back again. In the interests of safety, Phyllis had insisted and the boys had agreed to limit Don's and Jerome's driving shifts to no more than two hours. But once the gas gauge quit working, they recalibrated shifts to correspond to how far they could get on a tank of gas, estimated to be about 400 kilometres or four hours. Keeping to the spirit, if not the letter, of Phyllis's law would have to do. Much as they loved their mother, she would only get an edited version of the road trip that her sons were compelled to do in the heady summer of 1976. Which has much to do with what a road trip is all about.

The many challenges along the way, at least with the passage of time, are recounted as fun. Jerome remembers the journey to Lake Louise and the photo that was taken that is on the cover of this book. It was extremely hot, and as a swimming enthusiast, he started looking for a place to take a dip. Paul and Don decided to teach their brother about "shrinkage," decades before in an episode of *Seinfeld* the concept was enshrined into comedic mythology. Once the highway came parallel to the Bow River, the brothers magnanimously offered to stop and allow Jerome to cool off. Being a real swimmer, Jerome aggressively dove into the water, determined to swim across to the far shore. But the source of the Bow River is the Bow Glacier, which flows from the Rocky Mountains, and the temperature of the water tends to shrink both your perspective and your attached body parts. Jerome barely made it to the far shore and while still gasping for air was confronted with the fact that he had to re-submerge into the frigid water and swim back to his laughing brothers.

Jerome's affinity for water was particularly acute once they made it to within sight of the Pacific Ocean. They parked the van on a fairly steep hill, and Jerome decided to hike down to the water's edge and dip his feet into the water (he was careful not to immerse any other body parts). Don was somewhere else, so Paul sat in his wheelchair by himself with the brakes firmly locked while Jerome made his way to the shore. But being an adventurous type of guy, Paul reasoned that even with very limited hand dexterity, he could loosen his brakes just enough to allow for gentle progress down the hill towards the ocean.

When Jerome ascended to the van, he was puzzled that Paul, who could barely propel his wheelchair, was not in the spot where he had been carefully parked. Hurrying down the hill in a panic, Jerome saw an empty upturned wheelchair but, significantly, no sign of Paul. A quick search revealed that his brother had been thrown into a bush a disturbing distance away. Miraculously, Paul only had a few scratches and a slightly bruised ego. Mostly, the bobsled incident became fodder for laughter during the many hours of driving that were to come. Of course, part of the joke was that it was not the brakes of their decrepit van while descending mountains that became the *breaking* problem after all.

Today, modern customized accessible vans easily cost over $100,000 and are engineering marvels. Paul's old van was a small, depleted shell, the only nod to customized being a single sheet of plywood that was cut to fit the space where Paul slept each night crowded beside his snoring brothers. And to save their very limited funds, they intended to sleep, all three of them, all nights in the van. Even as brother Don explained the sleeping arrangements to me, I could not figure out how it worked, given that in addition to their belongings, Paul would need a wheelchair and considerable supplies in order to survive. Come to think of it, everything Don described—transfer into and out of the van, details of travelling with Paul, getting meals, brushing teeth, finding and using toilets, negotiating a million unforeseen obstacles and impossible barriers—was glossed over as *no big deal*—the same figure of speech Paul had used to describe the impossible decades earlier.

For example, I asked Don, "How in the world were you able to keep Paul clean on the road and in the heat of summer?" "Easy," Don responded (*No surprise*, I thought), "we went to cheap motels each week and negotiated a low price to borrow their shower for an hour." *Oh sure*, I thought, a proposal probably about as well received as a detective checking into Bates Motel. A few more logistical questions and more deflecting *no big deal* answers, and I finally said, leading to a bigger question, "Well, it would be a very big deal today, with far less obstacles and far better travelling vehicles for those few people willing to take it on; so how precisely was it no big deal to take on the impossible to make life an adventure in normal in those very early days of Paul's disability?" To which Don shrugged, at which time I realized that *no big deal* was less a deflection than an expression of love that is as close as unemotive brothers ever get to the inarticulate speech of their wounded hearts. And realizing this, I shut up. Actions shout; words whisper.

But of course, it was bloody extraordinary, a true miracle of communion, and although he hadn't said so when we talked, I could see the reflection of extraordinary in Don's eyes. The *no big deal* aspect of extraordinary was simply the absence of virtue signalling, credit seeking, and ego. Don had quit a promising job and promising career, and he and his wife moved back to Canada from Brazil where they were happy and had intended to stay, so that they could be close to Paul after they heard about his cancer. But shortly after they arrived, having dismantled their world without regret, Paul died. Don's career options would never be the same, but he and Jenny settled nicely in Atlantic Canada and opened a bed and breakfast, where he and I recently talked about Paul, 30 years after his death.

Jerome's *no big deal* devotion to Paul extended far beyond the infamous road trip. It is what I remember about Jerome when we first met. It is what Paul told me about his younger brother, and, consistent with who Paul was, he regarded that devotion with both appreciation and a cautionary note. Paul did not want his brother's altruism on his troubled path—even if he was a family member—to be the barrier to Jerome forging his own path. Don was like that, Jerome was like that, Paul was like that. Brothers can be like that.

Paul never did lose his sense of wonder. "How goes the battle?" was always an invitation to wonder, to comment on the adventure at hand, to solve what could be solved. Together. But on this day, in Paul's house, car dripping, feeling guilty as hell, I answered Paul's question. "I thought you just wanted me to come over to talk about something." My answer still rings hollow. Paul understood my predicament and instantly forgave me. The fact that he hadn't told me why he wanted me to come over doesn't mean I shouldn't have guessed. I shouldn't have been so easily forgiven, but the real lesson of forgiveness is that it is given regardless of our worthiness of it.

True friendship requires forgiveness. Talk to anyone about a long friendship gone sour, including or especially that friendship called marriage, and the reasons can often be distilled down to a failure to forgive. Paul was determined that his friendships not be about disability. The aneurism had happened to him, but it did not define him. Even being steeped in his own urine was external to who he was—unpleasant, but no big deal, and easily forgotten, instantly forgiven. There were more important issues in life for us to attend to, bigger battles to wage.

Such as work. Paul had landed at the Canadian Human Rights Commission, and each week we would strategize about how to move the needle on accessibility issues. Strictly speaking, we both worked on equity issues, but our approach, with his lead, was atypical of the time, completely out of sync with modern times. We instinctively ascribed to an active non-activist approach to activism—that is, doggedly and quietly pursuing real outcomes rather than the clatter of rhetorical intention, all noise and histrionics, outcomes being someone else's responsibility. Identifying problems and appropriating blame is the easy part; doing something about the problem, however imperfect, is what matters. When Paul asked, "How goes the battle?" he wanted a dispassionate account of possible outcome options, leading to an outcome achieved. He was not asking how I felt about it.

Decades later, Dr. John Meissner and I created a mental health program and conspicuously called it FITA: From Intention to Action, out of recognition that we all need a reminder that only in translating our good intentions into meaningful action can we move an issue, create change, and transform ourselves. Our intention must align with our higher self, doing what needs be done, making what is impossible today achievable tomorrow. Which might be an appropriate moment to insert a Winston Churchill quote that is as out of fashion today as the male mullet: "Sometimes doing your best is not enough. Sometimes you have to do what is required." World of difference.

What has been lost is the simple logic of Paul's well-lived life. First and foremost, Paul made people comfortable with him as a person, and because of this ability he was effective in advocating for accessibility issues on behalf of his constituents. It wasn't about him; it isn't about me; that is how real work is done. In evidence then, and increasingly today, the content of character and the uniqueness of the individual are regarded as less important than ubiquitous group interests.

There is both a logic and deep irony to the ascendancy of individual rights on the basis of membership in one's tribe. Logical, because if we, as a composite of physical features, are the temporary coming together of cells before oblivion, it makes sense to slug it out and contend for the survival of the fittest—that is, to contest for the power one derives from membership in the winning tribe. But it is ironic because the individual as understood and revered today did not exist until the advent of Christianity. And as the insignificant, square old conventional world of our ancestors is thrown off for chic modernity, it might be worth noting that the sanctity of the individual was the most radical epoch of thought the world had ever and has ever witnessed.

The world of antiquity through to the Romans when Christianity inexplicably sprang into being was brutal and barbaric in direct proportion to one's station, or caste, or to use a modern figure of speech, one's political identity. Slavery was not a result of being unassertive about one's human rights. One did not appeal to the United Nations if chosen for human sacrifice. Christianity was born into a world ruled by the absolute power of tyrants over the individual, most often expressed by cruelty, pain, and death. In the fourth century, Roman emperor Constantine actually became a Christian in acknowledgement of the fact that even the most powerful person in the world is subservient to another master. But this is not a God of another and higher tyrannical force; this God represents a doctrine of love, compassion, and the power of each individual soul's choosing to live forever, regardless of the temporal identity of human attributes.

The notion of elevating ourselves to our higher selves is more important today than ever. The modern obsession with individual rights (separate from the sanctity of the individual) and identity politics defines us by *what* we are to the exclusion of *who* we are and guarantees that we suffer. We will suffer from ME (modern ennui) syndrome—okay, so I made up the term, but since it spells "me," it seems appropriate. Living in the belief that this life is all there is leaves us fearful, and with a deep spiritual ache. Even the most committed atheist will acknowledge the existence of perpetual human longing, if only to herself. We ache for connection, we ache for fulfillment, we ache for love, we ache for what we cannot express. And even if we are able to avoid who we are with our many distractions during the light of the day, there is still waking from disquieting thoughts in darkness. Without distraction—a disquieting enough thought—stripped bare by splintered rumination that writhes and percolates, we are often afraid of the incoherent voice within us. Though disturbing, these moments may be our closest connection to who are, may be an opportunity to think deeply, beyond distraction and self-imposed limits of the material world, may be our first steps towards acknowledging and finding voice for the inarticulate speech of the heart.

Still, getting there is not easy. We all grow up in confusing times in large part because the act of growing up—if we opt for it—is confusing. And these are particularly confusing times for those actually trying to do so. We try to shield our kids from the world, snowplow away adversity, thereby stunting the necessary development of resilience. And for those whose parental mantra has been "the world is your oyster," this developmental delay can be painful.

I grew up in the 1960s—a tumultuous decade of change as well as the unfortunate advent of the "me" generation—but our brood of seven, most children of the boomer generation, escaped the worst aspects of the "me" revolution, which didn't stop us from inflicting them upon our children. Because however else our parents may have missed the parental mark, they at least spared us the burden of believing that life, this world, what meaning might exist, was all about us.

Increasingly, young people are brought up in the complete absence of spirituality. And if problems and questions arise, as they inevitably will, they have no basis, logic, or instinct for a spiritual life outside of, yet including, self. It is an interesting phenomenon that parents will work deliberately towards ensuring that their kids do not entertain any possibility of hope of life after death. Of course, the parental packaging of nihilism is couched in other socially accepted terms but tends to converge on the inflated notion of "self," which ironically is not only not the answer but may be the very problem. Unfortunately, post-COVID fear will exacerbate the sense of fragility that haunts young people immobilized by risk in the perpetually uncertain material world. With spirituality increasingly absent from people's lives even as mental health statistics worsen, the potential for finding a stabilizing anchor in the sea of uncertainty is diminishing.

I often think of Paul because his self-possession informs us 30 years later—that is, if we pay attention. Paul's comportment was certainly informed by his strong family ties and his practice of Catholicism, so I've lost most people already. Paul took pride in who he was and what he was able to accomplish as a person who happened to be a quadriplegic. He created meaningful change for persons with disabilities; he faced down with courage the many heartbreaking challenges of quadriplegia because of his admirable character. He did not, was unwilling to, lose his humanity in the details of his circumstances. To define ourselves by our various parts, our circumstances of birth, our good and bad luck, is to miss the opportunity for transcendence, to miss the whole, to deny the soul. The existence of our soul—a self-evident truth revealed by consciousness and demonstrated by character—is identity, that other apolitical identity, the one that does not die.

Paul's grace and courage remained intact until the end. In 1989, at age 37, Paul had some ailments, and after tests he was diagnosed with liver cancer. It was a death sentence. Though the life expectancy for quadriplegics had improved greatly by that time, they have to take harsh, invasive drugs, which cannot be healthy for the liver. Our livers are our filters, whose condition is determined by everything we have consumed in the past. The liver is to the body what history is to the human condition: it records the past, but the past is never past; it is where we find ourselves in the present and predicts the future.

The present we found ourselves in that day was Paul's hospital room moments after he matter-of-factly delivered the news. For the first time since we'd become friends, an awkward silence lay between us. The bulls**t of false hope was not possible, and so we hung suspended and without context. My eyes moist, my voice unsteady, he of dry eye and steady voice, we conversed some, though I don't remember a word either of us said. But I do know at some point he reassured me.

I could not respond about how I felt, what he meant to me, because once done it would be goodbye, and although the news was bad, it couldn't be time for goodbye.

Except that it was. Shortly after that visit he died, and although we felt deeply, it was a life lesson in the haunting power of the unspoken word. Still, I don't regret anything about that last meeting except that it was the last. I don't think we wanted last words—I know I wouldn't have. Weirdly, the problem of words unspoken can be negated by the heartbreaking concept of too painful for words. Guys seem particularly inept at emoting during pivotal moments and are sometimes better at establishing an unspoken understanding that is akin to intimacy. I realize that this statement comes across as disingenuous, considering the title and intent of this book. But it's my story, shared with Paul, and we're sticking to it. For now.

I missed our weekly conversations and felt lost without Paul's grounding context. Still, I got a chance a year later to gain back, if not conversations with Paul, increased conversations about him. The year Paul died, the province conceded that our work had value and provided funding to all universities in Ontario to establish a disability centre. Overnight, I went from measly me to a centre of four, and in January 1990, we opened the Paul Menton Centre for Students with Disabilities.

I was proud to have been able to entrench Paul's name into legacy, and students are still interested in knowing who he was. There is a nice story about Paul on our wall at the reception desk, but knowing who he was is another matter. On that first day, I remember feeling a glow from the unveiling of the centre in Paul's name, with the university president, dignitaries, and, most important, Paul's family in attendance. But I also had a vague feeling of being out of sorts, which I realized was the mild discomfort of having three new employees I didn't know what to do with. I'd been over seven years by myself in obscurity, and I think I resented the intrusion of outliers. It took me about five minutes to get to know, like, find work for, and be dependent on these, my peeps.

I have many great thoughts of Paul. He was funny, good company, easy to hang with. But in the mix, I also remember, and do not try to forget, the look on his face when we left his wedding early, or him looking at my dripping truck while sitting in his dripping pants. It isn't so much what I should have done (though regret hangs) as what I have learned, which is what a good friendship can teach. Memories of Paul are variously heartbreaking and joyous, and I don't want to dispel the bad any more than dwell in the good. The issue for me is less forgiveness than it is authenticity.

At this point, I probably should mention that I was a good and attentive friend to Paul. And if not for my Irish Catholic angst, I'd probably just go with that, and not sweat the seemingly minor transgressions. But that's not how I'm built, and perverse as it may seem, not how I want to be. I don't want to forgive myself, because I'm afraid I would then forget. I don't want to forget how bloody hard Paul's life was and how bloody miraculously he pulled it off until bloody hard became impossible, and he died. Paul literally lived his higher self, elevated his soul, even from the trajectory of sitting in a wheelchair in his own urine. It isn't what happens to us; it isn't the various parts we inherit, inhabit, or are left unfeelingly attached to after injury; it isn't karma or anything we did to deserve the cards we are dealt; "*it,*" as Van Morrison sings, "just is," and what we do with *it* is everything. Who we are, who we become, any meaning that has meaning, is about how we handle *it*, and in the subjugation of self for the eternal *it*, we elevate and glimpse into *soul*. It is where articulation and revelation become possible.

I can't do good without knowing I've done bad. I don't think guilt and conscience are archaic relics of a corrupt religious past. I will never have a moment of my higher self without knowing how bloody much I bottom dwell in my petty, small, physical world illusionary lower self. I need to stay grounded in order to hear the inarticulate speech from a thousand shouting hearts. They are there; I can feel them; I just can't quite hear them, yet.

Sometimes I think I'll meet Paul in the next life (though I'm not convinced I'm going to make it to his elevated habitat). He'll be standing—which I've never actually seen him do—with a cocky smile on his face, and he'll ask me, "How goes the battle?" and even though I'll want to tell him about all the extraordinary things that have happened since we last talked, I'll calm down and answer, "No big deal."

'Nough said. Talking is great, but the key to accessing the inarticulate speech of the heart exists in recognition. Through time, space, inevitable transformation, and hoped for revelation, he and I have seen and recognized each other.

Postscript: In rereading this chapter for a final edit I started thinking about Paul. Not a revelation, but late editing is more persnickety about details than concerned about content. I hadn't read the chapter in a while, and the blandness of mechanically rearranging words was pierced by the reality of Paul during that sweet spot in time of our early careers. We, me, all of us, live as if each day is simply a repeat performance of the one before, with others to continue as they always have without end. But seeing sameness is the complacent mind playing tricks. Look again, a little deeper, and when you see what is there, and when your mind stops creating what you assumed to be there, life's poignant, tragic, extraordinary—call it what you will—singularity will be revealed. I was thinking of Paul's singularity when the music on my ever-present Bluetooth speaker played "Last Train Home" by the Pat Metheny Group. It was playing on a tape cassette in my old Toyota 4 Runner moments after I learned from Paul that his prognosis was a death sentence, and for whatever reason it fixed onto my mind for these 30 years as emblematic of his crossing from this life to the next.

I don't think about Paul much anymore. It's been a while, and my mind has been cluttered by details and distractions, the shards of life that fill us up. Still, with the first few notes of "Last Train Home" Paul is back, my mind is uncluttered, there are no other people, and I am not limited by the illusion of sequential time. I think about where Paul's last train ended its journey and realize that the impenetrable cataclysm of death will be undone by our arrival home.

Chapter Three

EARLY TALES FROM THE ISLAND OF THE MISFITS

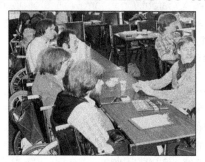

"One of the deepest longings of the human soul is to be seen."
John O'Donohue, Irish writer, Christian mystic (1956–2008)

Friends and acquaintances have often asked, "How the hell did you survive?" Meaning, how did a white, able-bodied, heterosexual, now middle-aged guy survive heading up an equity department in a university? Honest answer: I don't know. Simple answer: I tried to ignore the politics and focus on the people. Best answer, appropriated from Henry Kissinger, who after serving as secretary of state did a stint at Harvard whereupon he was quoted as saying, "University politics makes me pine for the relative peace of the Middle East."

Ignorance is not bliss; but for limited periods of time, it can be a blessing. Still, eventually you have to face the reality that your existence is sustained by ignorance. The fact is, we dwelt in that sweet spot before being politically awoken because nobody cared about our outlier issues and our little band of misfits, particularly me. As the issues, student numbers, and complexities grew, I could exit my foxhole, make a logical case, and wait to be ignored, or else hope for an institutional display of caring.

In my world—that solitary lair before the creation of the Paul Menton Centre for Students with Disabilities—there was no money, no real mandate, no hired help, just me and my obscure crew of students. We were at odds with how the world functioned—which also allowed us not to be limited by it—and for all that, my students were quite magnificent. The fight was for survival, and throughout the

1980s, I never heard the word *victim* from any of my students. It wasn't that people were not victimized, but once perception shifts from achieving a balance between systemic change and the bloody-minded need for *me* to change, *I am a victim* becomes the de facto mindset, and the ability to see the world as it is, is subverted to what you would have it be—always a formula for disillusionment, psychological pain, and bitterness. Yes, it was working with my little crew in those early, relatively apolitical years that saved me.

But no one could save me from Dennis. He was the first student I ever worked with, and after our initial slag-fest meeting he visited a couple of times a week for years. He was older, had been at university many years by then, and was looking for a place to call home. Apparently, my narrow slice of open corridor, relegated to status of office—being space nobody wanted in an institution where space is a more sought-after commodity than funding—fit Dennis's homing instinct bill. Apart from my charm and corridor/office combo, his other home, the one he had to get away from, was an empty apartment whose only visitors were paid attendants scheduled to visit twice each day to get him up in the morning and to return him to bed at night. There was no family, friends, or intimates to console, share a laugh with, or help answer the question, Who am I?

His daily repartee might begin with "How are you today, papist b*****d?" We had this Protestant versus Catholic thing going on, which even in the mid-1980s was out of date. It didn't actually require Dennis's opening salvo for me to know of his presence, since erratic driving of his electric wheelchair forewarned of his arrival. Inhabiting a slightly widened, unwanted corridor meant that I didn't have walls or a doorway to worry about scuffing. Dennis's speech was slow and slurred, so after training myself to understand him, I had to practice patience before replying, which I am really bad at. For that reason alone, I owe him.

It wasn't just that I had to resist finishing his sentences; I had to consider what he actually said, which was considerable. He was one bright guy whose intellect and daily passions were buried beneath people's impatience and unwillingness to listen. And of course, this double combo of others' impatience and indifference meant that he was terribly self-conscious. Our slagging routine—which, being Catholic and Irish, was perfectly up my alley—was a means to an end, the end being real conversation from an unexpected, rarely heard source.

If there is a silver lining to hardship, getting older, being uncool, and becoming invisible, it is this: it improves your conversational skills, allowing you to skip social convention, vacuous small talk, expectation, and frivolity for what matters, who matters, and what this short sojourn of living and dying might be about. Of course, I am frequently wrong and occasionally full of it, which has to be considered. I know because in addition to calling me a papist b*****d at the beginning and end of every conversation, Dennis told me so, just in case I took too seriously the real conversation we had just had. It was his way of divulging his deepest thoughts and fears without exposing too much vulnerability or leaving feelings on the table.

Long before doing and redoing a degree—completion oddly always two courses away—Dennis lived in the country with his grandmother. It was never explained what had happened to his parents, but it was very clear that life with his repressed and puritanical grandmother was antithetical to what a young person with a disability would need to thrive growing up. The prolonged university educational experience was pure liberation from the horror of his country experience, reminiscent of the iconic painting by Andrew Wyeth called *Christina's World*. In the painting, a young woman sits awkwardly in the foreground, looking back at her weather-beaten house. It is an American gothic, painted in 1948 during the great surge of optimism in post-war America. In that sense, it is not iconic of the age, but the image of isolation is emphasized by being separate from the great coming together everywhere else in the liberated world. Dennis's world mirrored Christina's world as a man out of time—his time, any time—a portrait of isolation.

Twenty years on and of indeterminate middle-aged, Dennis was encouraged/threatened by the prospect of graduating. Taking courses and building towards graduation had been a reason to get up in the morning, always with a vague notion of application in the working world outside of post-secondary la la land. But between the papist b*****d opening and closing remarks of each encounter, during the time of real conversation, he would ask, though pleading would be a more accurate descriptive, "Do you think I could ever get a job?"

I'm told I can be disarmingly honest, which is to say I can be harsh. I don't know if it is my Depression era Second World War graduate parents or my middle position in the muddle of seven children, but saying niceties to placate people has never been possible for me. This is especially true if I respect people, and I liked and respected Dennis. So, I couldn't tell Dennis that yes, of course, a career in accounting starting at six figures is waiting for you the moment you graduate. I also did not articulate the stark reality of which he was fully aware. I really didn't know, though I knew he was in tough. I also suspected that he was not even sure if he wanted a career as an accountant, but he would have liked some respect. He deserved that, but it is well-known in the accessibility business that an attitude change is a much tougher gig than building ramps or funding services. Everyone just assumes that their attitude is the most enlightened in the world, for no particular reason. But most people do not, never did, see Dennis.

• • •

Bill's face had a funny quality. It was analogous to my dog Zigo's perpetual wagging tail. Bill's face constantly registered a smile, but it was not just an expression of his mouth and lips. His face erupted into a contorted glow, all teeth, happiness, and goodwill. Bill's hair turned almost white while he was still in his twenties, but that fact didn't really age him. Or if it did give him a slight air of distinction, he reverted back to a teenager whenever he flapped his gums and revealed a smile that could win over anyone for any reason. Bill was easygoing and easy to like.

He was a hanger-on from among the first wave of quadriplegics who had muscled their way into the residence before it was equipped to qualify as habitable during the 1970s. Some of the early group had graduated; many did not. Bill was the last to neither admit defeat nor be defeated. He just hung around and hung on. He, like Dennis, like many others, didn't know what else to do.

It was with Bill in mind that the housing department changed its residence policy that required students to take a full course load. The policy change had intended to entrench the reality that students with high-level physical disabilities might need more time to complete a degree. The policy change was necessary and came from a good place but also gave people like Bill—well, actually there was no one like Bill—permission to take as much time as they wanted. Bill wanted all the time in the world.

In addition to buildings, classrooms, and residence rooms that were inaccessible, students requiring attendant service were stranded between getting up in the morning and going to bed at night. And because residence life included fun-loving, rollicking activities and spontaneous parties—with students with disabilities joining in—the span of hours between getting up and going to bed were many and unpredictable. The idea could have been to allow students with disabilities the freedom and independence of other students, but it would be more accurate to say that no one was paying attention. And problems developed. Instructing drunken buddies with alcohol-induced slurred speech on how to get you into bed at 3 a.m. long after attendants have gone home is not a winning formula. In those circumstances, the hoped for safe and careful transfer of a vulnerable person really was just throwing someone into bed without much thought about how he landed. Then again, that was also the age when students smoked most anywhere and people didn't much wear seatbelts. Fun times.

Dr. Mary O'Brien, director of health services, took note, and a nursing satellite office was opened in residence to help prevent students from being stranded. The nurses worked hard and did their best for these pioneers of university life, but they were outnumbered and were no match for the immensity of the challenge. At the same time, the housing department acknowledged that students with disabilities had to fight with their rooms and undertook to do the first retrofitting aimed at enhancing accessibility. These were important first steps, an honest acknowledgement of a problem, which is always the necessary precursor to finding a solution. I was reminded of feisty Dr. O'Brien—whose accent persisted some 70 years after leaving Scotland—when reading that she died on May 5, 2020, age 95. Most of all I remember and am grateful to Dr. O'Brien because she did not recoil from allowing me to attack persistent problems with bold, if occasionally wacky, solutions.

Straying outside of convention—rather than continuing along the path of least resistance—I came up with a plan and got lucky. No, not in the young, wild students-in-residence sense, but with a solution to the attendant services issue. Students with disabilities were given limited individual needs-based funding through a program called Vocational Rehabilitation Services. VRS had given a one-time contribution to the first rudimentary renovations in residence. Though VRS was emphatic that this one-time contribution was in no way precedent setting—from individual to collective funding—I questioned the sense of that claim. Students needed twenty-four-hour attendant service, but since they were funded for a piecemeal system of individual attendants coming twice a day to serve individuals, students spent long hours waiting for help. It was also inefficient and expensive, managed by a private company that took a cut, whose employees were paid for a minimal number of hours each time they came, and with a ton of transportation issues for attendants within this split-shift mayhem.

I did the math, and in a two-page proposal I argued that with a modest increase we could create a twenty-four-hours-a-day seven-days-a-week system out of the ashes of our piecemeal junk by hiring our own trained students living in residence, thereby eliminating travel costs, high hourly rates, and the private company take. In addition to addressing the stranded student issue, in time we could expand service to helping with mealtime, a perpetually difficult issue for students. (Note of acknowledgement: For two years before funding arrived, based on a one-time comment to Ray Klassen, the Navigators volunteered for all meals for our students seven days a week.)

I willed myself to forget about the proposal the day I submitted it. Which may be why I received a response a couple of weeks later and had funding in place the following month. I suspect that governments at all levels have become less responsive, less susceptible to common sense, deferring to experts and policy wonks for whom the dictates of responsiveness and common sense are no longer relevant. Same for getting institutional permission to submit a proposal for a program, for a service, for an idea that has never been done. But, as previously confessed, I can be harsh or, put another way, I had low tolerance for virtue signalling long before it was named and became a thing.

Once we received funding, I just assumed that other post-secondary institutions would apply for and receive the same. And yet, the attendant service program is still the only twenty-four-hours-a-day seven-days-a-week 365-days-a-year program embedded in university residence in the world. In later years, we expanded attendant services into the residence of our sister college across town, and that too was, and is likely, the only 24-7 program in a college residence in the world.

We always wondered why our program remained singular. And then the answer was unspectacularly revealed in a phone call from the minister's office. That would be the same minister's office that had funded our program for these past three decades and counting. The minister's office asked a troubling question: "Why does the attendant service program only exist at your university?" *Good question*, I thought, *but a bit weird coming from the funding ministry*. Still, it is not unusual for governments to fund programs without understanding why. So as delicately as I could—and reminding myself that now is not the time to be harsh—I asked a few questions. Apparently, the mother of a quadriplegic had asked why attendant services were not available in their northern Ontario hometown university, and ministry people were in a panic to provide an answer to this demanding mother.

She was not demanding, or, better put, she and her son had lots of skin in the game and had every right to be demanding, assertive, or whatever label fits. The sad truth is, unless a campus has the basic accessible infrastructure so that students can move independently around campus, there won't be any students who would need attendant service. Too often in life problems are ignored so that they can go away. Accessibility is not an impossibility but tends not to be what universities compete to do. Solutions are there in our grasp if we squeeze hard. It is a matter of commitment, proper sequence, and—sorry for multiple use of the term—common sense. Oh yeah, and doing what you said you were going to do.

In those early years, accessibility was not much understood. Higher learning does not necessarily correlate with much understanding. Still, I liked outlier perspective—able to get things done without outside interest or interference—even if that meant little support. And outlier status occasionally resulted in real humour. One day I received a rare—well, first time—call from the president's office. Our university had been informed that it had won the 1987 Ontario Minister's Special Award for Excellence in Creating a Barrier Free Environment.

This prestigious award was given out each year by the minister for the Office of Disabled Persons in acknowledgement of new accessible architecture that exceeded building code standards. The president and the director of architecture were going to Toronto the next day to receive the award, and without acknowledging that I was an afterthought, they asked if I could join them. Our limo ride to the airport was chatty, that is between the president and the director of architecture. Not being included in chattiness, I had time to wonder. Our buildings were not exemplars of accessibility, and, more to the point, there had not been any new buildings constructed or significant renovations completed in recent years.

Once we arrived in Toronto, we were seated at the very front of the assembled crowd. Chattiness continued until the minister spoke. He briefly outlined the history of the award before adding that in this one year, it was being given to our attendant service program for innovation in programming, rather than for architectural accessibility. It was never said, but I'm fairly certain that neither the president nor the director of architecture had any idea of the existence of the attendant service program.

There are moments in our life that are captured in perpetuity, not unlike romantic poet John Keats's "Ode on a Grecian Urn." I was grateful that in their bewilderment, neither the president nor the director of architecture glanced in my direction. I fear that they might have discerned the trace of a smile. It wasn't smugness, just a realization of possibility. The rest of the award ceremony is a forgettable blur, but I do remember the limo ride back to the airport being distinctly unchatty. I was grateful that no questions were asked, no congratulations offered.

Despite the dark mood, I suspect there was a discernible glow from the corner of the limo where I sat. It was not my victory; it was subversive articulation, an intimacy we misfits shared shrouded in our cloak of invisibility. We had been acknowledged as exemplars by a provincial minister, and I could envision the president the next day searching a university directory to figure out just where these outliers were located.

For most of Bill's many years at university he struggled. In addition to having to deal with limited accessibility, he chose, as many quadriplegics do in the early years, to use a manual wheelchair. This is a commitment to a difficult physical regime, a deliberate refusal to capitulate to the electric wheelchair, after which there is no returning to the manual chair. It is, if only symbolically, the last physical piece of self to have to give up in the zero-sum dance towards very limited mobility. But propelling a manual wheelchair for a quadriplegic is slow, painfully slow, and difficult—continuously rolling a boulder uphill seems a fitting comparison. The one big fortuitous but unintended advantage we had over other northern campuses was an elaborate underground tunnel system connecting all buildings. The tunnel system made getting to all buildings possible in all weather, though the distances were great, which did not stop Bill from embracing the struggle those few times he actually went to class. His night life required that he sleep in late, so there was no spotting Bill en route to morning classes. But astonishingly, when a late afternoon Bill-spotting occurred, he always framed the picture of painstakingly negotiating his manual chair with a big, impossibly big, smile. Later, when he was placed in a newly renovated semi-accessible room with access to attendant service at his odd-hour discretion, Bill said he felt like a king. He wasn't serious, though he said so with a smile on his face. It was one more reason to delay departure from the residence, his home.

Bill thought that the story of his accident, the one that permanently made him into a quadriplegic, was funny. One might think that Bill thinking the story of his accident funny was weird. Recalling details of the event must have been traumatic, but he may have needed to reframe trauma into humour in order to cope. Not sure, but the way he and others have magnificently pulled a life from the ashes of incomprehensible loss requires that we listen. It's easy to translate *we laugh so as not to cry* as denial. Still, maybe there's a place for denial in our eerily uncertain cataclysmic lives, punctuated by the certainty of loss.

The way Bill told the story was funny enough, but it was also easy to see the human beneath the humour. He had fatalistic charm; he communicated more with a shrug of the shoulder—limited by paralysis—than most of us could communicate in a lifetime as an auctioneer. The humour was that his accident was caused by his van hitting a cow—that's right, a milking moo moo. In Newfoundland, the number one cause of vehicle death and serious injury is from encounters with moose. Seems so much more dignified somehow. But a cow? That is funny, at least the way Bill told it. The human beneath it all was that the freak encounter with a large animal—it is physics after all and not animal status that determines extent of damage—robbed

Bill of that other life, the one denied, the people he might have known, the places he might have visited, the great love of his life he didn't have, that child or six who were not born, that other life not talked of or joked about, *the other*. These are not healthy thoughts, but how do you not have them? Tell funny stories. These unfunny thoughts were not evident in his smile. We all lie to survive, and sometimes a lie is really just a pleasing way to package naked courage.

And yet as I reflect back on Bill's impossibly big smile, something else has to be considered. Someone outside of another's experience might presumptuously interpret difficulties as impossible to live with. Still, many people find a version of happiness—focusing on what they have and letting go of what they have lost—whatever life's vicissitudes, some even after being dealt the queen of spades. Maybe inability to not understand someone's experience should evoke neither puzzlement nor judgment. Maybe we should instead wonder at the appearance of common among individuals who pull themselves into their higher selves from wherever they find themselves in life.

Bill liked to hold events. He didn't want to actually organize them, but he was open to others succumbing to his will. When I was new to my job, I was looking for some way to make inroads with the residence gang, so it was the perfect match. He wanted to organize a wheelchair basketball game that included members of the men's national wheelchair basketball team. We asked our men's basketball team to sit in a wheelchair for an hour against a group of people who resided in one. Wheelchair basketball can be a real rough and physical game, and it takes skill and strength. Our talented varsity basketball team didn't quite believe how much grit and talent was required until they were given a reality lesson. They lost in spectacular fashion, but for those familiar with wheelchair basketball it was not a surprise. Try controlling a basketball while negotiating a wheelchair, then try shooting a ball from said chair, close up at first, and then from a distance. Watch said basketball drop miles in front of the desired target.

While the outcome of the game was predictable, the outcome of the unstated main event was very much in doubt. Basketball was the prelude to the raffle, the main event and a residence life custom of some years. All week residence houses competed to sell the most raffle tickets for a 40-ouncer of Southern Comfort. What the raffle was raising funds for was never revealed, and there must be 100 reasons why this event could not be held on any university campus today.

I still think of Bill when I hear mention of an anti-alcohol policy, or anti-whatever, *anti* being what policies are designed for today. I picture Bill smiling, half shrugging, and saying, "Who, me?" He would never have admitted to it, but Bill gave me the traction to make the connection with the people who I needed to connect with to grow a part-time job into a vocation.

He eventually did graduate, so he had to leave, and we lost contact. Like so many of these guys, they were all there until they were gone. At some distant point after his departure, I learned that Bill had died while still young. Today he would smile and think me rather pathetic for trying to figure out meaning, death, spirituality, and the like without making a joke. He might think how humorous it all is, how off the mark I am for making complex out of the simplicity of a big smile and an innocent shrug of the shoulders. And in a funny kind of way, he is probably right.

• • •

The most memorable image I have of another Paul of my experience is not his physical form but his impeccable handwriting. I am choosing the word *hand* rather than *cursive* writing deliberately. Message neatly and conscientiously written down on a sheet of paper and carefully placed beside my phone, content long forgotten, though I do remember being impressed at the time by his attention to detail. He did not work for me, he was not a volunteer, but he had taken a message, the proof being his handwritten note. Still, I stood looking down at his handiwork forever long, marvelling at the fantastical nature of commonplace revealed.

Paul did not have hands or arms, feet or legs. What Paul had was consideration, a desire to contribute, and adaptive skills that are still hard to believe. Paul was one of my early students and one of over 1,200 babies born in Europe, Canada, and Japan with severe congenital defects as a result of their mothers taking the drug thalidomide during pregnancy. In the late 1950s, some mothers were prescribed thalidomide to help with morning sickness. This was during a time of great optimism and innocence when people did what their doctors ordered without question. Morning sickness can be very unpleasant, but no one had ever died of it. Still, the post-war era sought convenience in a way the pre-war generation could not have imagined. Whether treated or not, the effects of morning sickness are short-lived, but the effects of thalidomide treatment for morning sickness continue to this day.

In 1957, a German pharmaceutical company called Chemie Grunenthal produced the drug and distributed it to 46 countries. The drug had known side effects. Thalidomide caused peripheral neuropathy or numbness of hands and feet, but not to be deterred, Chemie Grunenthal marketed the drug as "completely non-poisonous." And to the mothers coping with morning sickness, apart from numbness, the drug was true to its marketing claim. But to their fetuses, to the tiny human beings whose emerging existence caused their mothers' morning sickness, thalidomide delivered irreparable cataclysmic damage, not to life but certainly to limb.

By the narrowest of margin due to the power of one, the drug never made it into the giant U.S. market. In 1960, the Federal Drug Administration refused to approve thalidomide based on the expertise or fortuitous hunch of Dr. Francis Kelsey. To the benefit of American consumers, Dr. Kelsey continued working for the FDA into her 80s.

By 1959 in Europe, where thalidomide first became available, babies began being born with "flipper limbs" in epidemic proportions. Still, the connection to thalidomide was not made until 1961, and remarkably it was not pulled from distribution in Canada until March 1962. For Paul and his family, bad luck was to follow upon negligence, incompetence, and criminal responsibility. Paul's mother had inadvertently kept thalidomide pills long after they had been banned in Canada. Paul was born in May 1964, so sometime late in 1963 Paul's mother took the banned pills and innocently changed the lives of an incalculable number of people. As removed as I am from the important people in Paul's life, and further removed by almost 60 years since the taking, I count myself among them. Such is the unforeseen power of connection.

Long before Paul became my student, long before Paul impressed me with the miracle of his phone skills and handwriting, I knew of Paul before I knew he was Paul. I knew of him from a distance, on the street, passing his house twice daily on my way to and from my first year of high school. And I wondered.

I hated school, always had trouble sitting all day, spent distracted hours looking outside the classroom window for a sprig of green or a glimpse of blue, wanting to be anywhere else than in class. The need and ability to move goes a long way towards explaining my many warts and desires, so absolutely my first thoughts about Paul were about perspective and yes, gratitude. I felt sympathy for him and was glad I was not him. I also felt ashamed for seeing Paul without really seeing him (for that takes knowing him). Each morning at the same time, a taxi arrived, and a driver first carried Paul to the car and then went back to the house for what must have passed as a Stalinist version of legs—a frightening wooden abomination, equal parts utilitarian structure and symbol of immobility. Presumably he was placed into the cavity of the structure to replicate the act of standing. I hadn't known that such a device was possible, same for the phenomenon of what I was later to learn was Paul. The terrible thing was not what Paul was but the fear people felt who regarded him as outside of what it is to be human. Far too much for a child to have to deal with, and yet he did just that.

The effect of thalidomide on Paul was particularly severe. Three limbs completely missing, with one very short, and in its solitary configuration a particularly useful stump of no more than six inches long. It was under his wristwatch band on his one stump that Paul was able to place a pen with his very dexterous mouth, which allowed him to take my phone message, and it was both a marvel to behold and no big deal to see.

I don't remember Paul ever looking up at me as he was carried to the taxi. I'm glad. The look on my face would not have conveyed friendliness. It was likely an all too familiar portrait of what my mother would have called gawking. Gawking and fear equal distance. I'm glad Paul knew me later when he learned to quell fear by simply being comfortable with himself, allowing gawkers to step back into the distance and disappear into the woodwork of their sheltered lives.

Paul's taxi ride to school may have been the highlight of his day, particularly since he was assigned to the handicapped unit, a mishmash of students with physical and psychiatric disabilities as well as students with behavioural problems. It was the school board's *island of the misfits*, designed to protect mainstream students rather than provide appropriate education to students with specific needs. These early "special education" forays were not kind to those whose specific need was to get an education. Part of Paul's problem was that he was very bright and he genuinely wanted to learn. The handicapped unit had many continuous distractions from learning in addition to profound social isolation in the midst of a gawking crowd. Paul's other problem was that he was very social.

When our attendant service program ramped up to 24 hours in the mid-1980s, we had more students with high levels of physical disabilities living in the energetic cauldron of partying and social jostling of residence life. Many of our students with disabilities grew up in small towns, where social interaction did not much exist. Many of the able-bodied students had grown up indifferent to or perhaps gawking at the few people with disabilities they had ever encountered. But for better or for worse, residence life is the great mixer of people from disparate parts of life, and whatever social coagulation happens, happens. And what happened, and what still happens, is that mostly people work it out, and mostly it works out fine. Lots of unavoidable exposure and interaction, many friendships, a bridge from segregation to the real world—messy as it sometimes is. Rarely is social isolation better than engagement.

I was a very poor student. In my school we had an "opportunity" class, which everyone knew was a euphemism for "dummy" class. This was almost ten years before Paul's handicapped "opportunity," and it terrified me the same way we ignorantly understood the experience of being a leper or a "retard." For years, I feared that I would be called into the principal's office and told that I had been selected for opportunity status.

It is impossible to know what it cost Paul in his early years to persevere on the island of the misfits. The great cruelty that kids are capable of most commonly happens when one kid is isolated from the pack. Just how do you negotiate your existence when your mere physical presence disturbs the kids you are trapped with who are themselves disturbed? How do you present who you are to people who have no understanding of who anyone is? In Paul's handicapped school one student shrieked uncontrollably every time he saw him. Most disturbing is that senior school board officials who never stepped foot inside this classroom thought that these two students belonged together.

Paul could not endure the shrieks. It remains unknown how long the shrieker could have continued his daily barrage. No solution was offered, so Paul had to leave. For three months, he stayed at home while his parents searched for a school that would take him. Maybe it was during this time that Paul became motivated to learn on his own. He mostly taught himself French, Arabic, German, and at university, Italian. Five languages including English is impressive enough, but it gets better. Paul taught himself to write—an adaptation extraordinaire—at age five.

The not-so-silent shriek that ended Paul's tenure at the handicapped school worked out well. This is where exposure to people helps all concerned—even or especially for those at the tender age of 13. After his prolonged timeout, Paul was warmly welcomed by Sister Eleanor Hennessy at St. Brigid's School. St. Brigid's did not have a handicapped class, and Paul was in a regular setting, which was a significant improvement. Still, he was used to being excluded from school activities—especially from anything remotely fun. But when St. Brigid's had an outdoor winter event, Paul's habitual exclusion was overturned, and he was taken tobogganing.

Today, schools are often immobilized from taking kids on field trips or allowing any activity with a sniff of fun out of a frenzied fear of, well, everything. Risk aversion at all costs out of a societal need to cover its collective a*s does not make for a good education and may be contributing to our kids' mental illness. Kids need to explore, be confronted with adversity, and the resultant resilience in doing so is their best defence against fragile mental health.

For Paul, isolated by way of attachment to a crude immoveable contraption ironically called legs, the thrill of racing down a wintery slope attended to and the centre of a classmate's attention would have been an epoch of liberation. He may have felt some fear, but that is the price of a thrill, and this was the thrill of a lifetime. The excitement of movement without control and his own shrieks of laughter likely deafened the shrieks from his former handicapped life. Paul hungered for experience in his life, searching for ways to transcend his physical condition, even as he accepted the cards he was dealt. Much later in life, he said, "I think able-bodied. I even dream able-bodied." It is easy to take mobility for granted. It is possible to both accept one's condition and hunger for something completely outside one's experience.

No doubt it was the hunger that drove him to go skydiving. Seems to be the epitome of vulnerability, though I suppose having limbs isn't going to help much if the parachute doesn't open. Taking risks and mixing it up with people having fun is a good defence against vulnerability and the one that matters most, social isolation. Paul knew that.

At university he thrived. Paul's Italian professor, Claudia Persi Haines, department chair and friend, said he was *the* best student, not just of that course or year but her all-time career best. Since he was young, Paul had wanted to become a translator, and his ambition was matched by his talent. But this ambition was in conflict with another. He wanted to travel, and he wanted to escape Canadian winter—the hardship of which is greatly exacerbated by the need for a wheelchair.

Both bad and good things happen when least expected. Paul's twenty-year pending case was settled. Paul's law firm had finally won his case against the makers of the thalidomide drug, and he was rich. After which, Paul travelled the world and escaped hellish winter. And as often happened with my students, we lost contact.

Until, three years after the fact, I read about Paul's death on February 22, 2016, at age 51. I learned that he had not simply sailed to a southern location never to be found. Money had given him some freedom to move long distances, but it had not freed him of thalidomide. In university, he had not wanted to be an activist. Paul had wanted to make his mark unconnected to his physical circumstances. He liked people, and he studied languages, and who doesn't want to converse with someone in five languages?

I then came across a photo of Paul on December 2, 2014, just after 256 members of Parliament stood in unanimous acknowledgement of Canada's responsibility to thalidomide victims, fully 50 years after the fact. The acknowledgement included a settlement to victims—not like Paul's legal settlement, but something, an acknowledgement of thalidomide's destructive continuing effects and, most important, that victims were not responsible. Another photo showed Paul typing a message on his smart phone—requiring almost as much dexterity as answering my phone 30 years earlier—with his stump, mouth, and shoulder working in perfect harmony.

Despite becoming rich, Paul had become an activist after all. He had become the vice-president of the Thalidomide Victims Association of Canada at a time when another important issue was emerging. Even after its horrible recent history, thalidomide was making a comeback. It had been used as a treatment for leprosy sores in the past but had even more relevant modern applications for treatment of cancer, blindness, and especially AIDS. A biotech company called Celgene was looking to reintroduce the drug, albeit under conditions that would make it the most regulated drug in the world. Though there was no risk of thalidomide's history repeating itself, the Thalidomide Victims Association had good reason to oppose reintroduction of the drug. Still, on behalf of the association, Paul saw an opportunity to advance the cause with dollars and issued a practical proclamation as he asked for one million dollars. "If we are going to allow this to happen, then we expect something in return. It's a business transaction."

Paul's practical opportunism should not have been a surprise. He was neither immobilized by nor embittered by his condition. So he, who no longer needed money, went out and got money for the continuing cause, a casual example of leadership and courage that he would have regarded as anything but.

In all my years working with persons with disabilities, I have learned astonishing little. Well, I've learned lots of stuff, but I have not penetrated anyone's experience, from which learning that matters most happens. I wish I had wisdom or insight, as some people assume, into Paul or Chris or Bill, but I don't. It isn't for lack of trying; it isn't that I haven't tried to be there in that place of understanding—more to the point, I am nowhere, except perhaps in wonder. For all the instantaneous and frequent communication of the world today, we are locked out of each other's essential experience, the core of our personhood, our invisible, silent, all-pervasive screaming consciousness.

Still, for all I don't know, I know this. It isn't just crossing the threshold to passive acceptance or learning how to finally cope or burying the past because it is dead and gone or embracing one's new reality, whatever that is. For all that is involved with making a profound psychological shift—and that is huge—there is always that not insignificant detail about applying the same every minute of every hour, day in, day out, for a long as there are days to repeat. This application, that courageous effervescence, is not static but is a task of perpetual, astonishingly difficult, motion.

Whenever my friend Paul, the other one whom we named our centre after, began our weekly conversation with the question "How goes the battle?" he was only being mildly facetious. Life is a battle that we don't win. But if there is a soul—and the various Pauls of my experience convince me that there is—it comes to the surface in the wonder we feel in the absence of understanding. The two Pauls fill me with wonder, and the absence of wonder in life is *a-Pauling*. An appalling pun, I know, but the Pauls of my life would appreciate and understand. It was the frivolous way we articulated what is buried deepest and matters most.

Chapter Four

ANGEL EYES

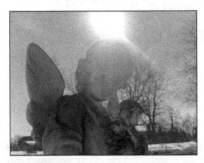

"And every guy has got you in his sight
What you're doing with a clown like me
Is surely one of life's little mysteries."
"Angel Eyes," from album *See the Light,* The Jeff Healey Band, 1988

If, as philosopher Pascal Blais said in the seventeenth century, "all man's miseries derive from not being able to sit in a quiet room alone," what happens if you are consigned to sit in a quiet room alone without experience or sight to give context or means of expression? What if beneath enforced quiet rages an inarticulate speech of the heart that cannot be quailed by personal circumstance? What if one has to *do* in order to *be*?

I met Jeff Healey once, but I didn't know him. Still, anyone who had any exposure to him knew he was about music. Music made him famous, but it was more than just that. From early on until his early death, Jeff Healey navigated the world, formed relationships, and articulated what he wanted known through an astonishing width and breadth of musical expression. He inhaled oxygen; he exhaled music.

Cara, who likes to better me as my better half, hears that I once met Jeff Healey and one-ups me with "Oh yeah, well, I went to school with him at Etobicoke Collegiate Institute," "We were in the same class," "We talked together," and "I sat beside him at the piano." She would go on if not for the incredulity registering on my face. This makes her happy. Cara says I'm hard to impress, and clearly, I'm impressed. After I query why she has never told me about this fascinating aspect of her life, I ask, "What was he like?" as she counters with "How did you meet him?"

Being the better half, first Cara: "He was incredible. He sang, played the piano, the guitar, talked about music, seemed to know everything about music; he was a real sweetheart."

"So, the rumour he was discovered by Stevie Ray Vaughan is not true because of the earlier discovery made by you."

I try to make this sound pathetically poetic. Being married to me, Cara is allowed to selectively ignore me with impunity, so I continue. "Easy to talk to?"

"Very. Very personable, and he had sex appeal too." That answer was unsolicited.

"High school is not exactly an easy place to be different. How was he regarded by other students?"

Cara thinks about this. "There were always the clowns and a**holes who would pin themselves against their lockers when he walked down the corridor with his white cane, but mostly he seemed cool and comfortable with himself, and as far as I could tell he fit in well."

"And he didn't have a guide dog?"

"No, I never really thought about it then; probably because he always seemed know where he was going, down the corridor and in life." Cara stops suddenly with a need-to-know exclamation, which she does several times each wondrous day. "How is it possible to get around in a visual world if you are blind? And I remember sitting beside him, watching him play the piano, wondering how in the world could he play so well? The piano is a big instrument, and to play well, you have to move your hands quickly and accurately to notes that are far apart. He never seemed to make a mistake, which I can't do even playing pieces I know well. And he played the guitar on his lap like it was a keyboard. Have you ever seen him play the guitar? He also played other instruments, probably perfectly. How is any of this possible?"

I think about my students these 35 years on, how they cope, manage, thrive, how they negotiate their life, this world; the average, innocuous, unseen, unheroic, and unsung; and then those who astound, including but not limited to Jeff Healey, one of the truly great singers, songwriters, musicians, musicologists, broadcasters, and—in consideration of music that only came to light years after his death—a Lazarus-like creative force such as the world has never seen before and may never see again—and I answer, "I have no idea."

Still, I am impressed that she homed in on *the* central question on my mind all these years. How is the ever-expanding *it* possible? Since I don't, can't, answer, Cara persists in a cloud of protest as my mind travels back through the years. She doesn't expect me to dissect or shed light into the phenomenology of Jeff Healey's many accomplishments, but she is unsatisfied that I cannot offer any insight into the basic question regarding how a person without sight—surely the fundamental tool needed to way-find, play the piano, pound with perfection his trademark guitar—can soar, quite possibly surpassing all full-sighted human accomplishment. I disappoint people on this question on a regular basis despite my many years of pondering. I could give some trite mechanical information that would serve to obscure or explain away rather than offering anything of any depth. No amount of mechanical functioning explains essence, drive, or genius. Jeff Healey was a musical genius whose drive and essence remain a mystery. And being older now, and not married to material-world thinking (being married to Cara instead), I am comfortable not knowing the answer to most of life's many imponderables. I just am. Questions—continuing with the marriage analogy—coupled with wonder are enough. Besides, what would we do if we had it all figured out? Life is far more interesting for what we don't know than what we do. And in the one-up(wo)manship marriage that we have, I enjoy frustrating Cara with what she thinks I know but will not say. I also enjoy her not knowing how little I actually know.

Now, back to that one time I met Jeff Healey. In 1990, with the Paul Menton Centre well on its way, we began working with the student government on accessibility issues. Student government wonks tend to be distrustful of the big bad university administration folks, and though I looked student-esque, I was, at least officially, on the big bad side. Still, between the student government and the university administration, we managed to create a fund to deal with physical accessibility issues. Possibly a historical first, and 30 years later the cost-sharing arrangement continues without murder or mayhem.

As a consequence, in 1991 the student government decided they wanted to have their own award for an accomplished student with a disability. To give the award some muscle, they wanted to launch it in the name of someone of stature. At the time, The Jeff Healey Band was huge in Canada and far beyond. In addition to major accolades earned in rapid succession around this time, Jeff Healey starred as Patrick Swayze's long-time pal in a terrible, yet in retrospect an oddly cult-like, film called *Roadhouse*. The film is late 1980s' cheesy extraordinaire, every scene and line of dialogue predictable and fake. Your film review could succinctly summarize it as a sequence of glaring gender stereotypes, big hair, and any excuse for Patrick Swayze to take off his shirt. And yet there is a slight redemptive quality from the great and authentic music courtesy of the Roadhouse band, played by the Jeff Healey Band. Jeff has a few lines with pal Patrick as well, and his deep voice and comportment give the film some much needed maturity from the unlikely 23-year-old blues rocker.

The Jeff Healey Band's 1988 debut album *See the Light* went platinum in the giant U.S. market and triple platinum in Canada. The cut "Hideaway" from that album was nominated for a Grammy for Best Rock Instrumental Performance, which was acknowledgement of Jeff Healey's inclusion into the rarified club of world's best guitarists. In 1990, he won a Juno Award as Best Canadian Entertainer of the Year. Also, in 1990, he covered George Harrison's "While My Guitar Gently Weeps," with George Harrison and Jeff Lynne on backup vocals and acoustic guitar! But why be satisfied collaborating with only one Beatle? Jeff Healey was invited to join Ringo Starr and His All-Starr Band, a rotating group of the very best musicians in the world. I'm ashamed to admit it, but I didn't know any of these specifics when we met, only the general swirl of Jeff Healey's emerging fame. One day at a meeting with discussion about a mysterious larger than life figure who could front the award, I suggested Jeff Healey, which was swatted down, he being big, but too big. "But, but, but ..." I stammered, "why not ask and see what happens?"

What happened was he said yes to creating the award in his name, and shockingly, weeks later he turned up in person to help launch the Jeff Healey Award for Students with Disabilities. Which was both a surprise and huge embarrassment. I hadn't made the phone call to ask Jeff to let his name stand, and I hadn't asked him to come. Someone in the student government had managed to contact Jeff Healey, got him to agree to let his name stand for the award, and even convinced him to come to the event. Presumably that mysterious student government person had made all the arrangements, since it was their event, and involvement from our centre would not have been welcome. But as Jeff entered the gymnasium and stood awkwardly at the entrance with his parents, with no one from the student government moving to greet him, it became clear that no arrangements had been made. In fact, I never could get anyone to even admit that Jeff Healey had been asked.

It is a moment frozen in time. He who ruled the rock and blues world, with a whole other tsunami of jazz talent on the horizon, timidly stood, unseen, unseeing, and unknown, in a world in which he had become extremely well-known—just ask George Harrison. His parents were directly behind, close by but not taking over the situation that was Jeff's to negotiate, as was likely their lifetime habit. This balance between heartfelt support and the necessity of autonomy and independence is the painful and delicate tightrope that is the life of parents of a kid with a disability, including an adult rock star. Heartache and restraint, the delicate parental balancing act, always.

Jeff had been adopted when he was a baby and lost one eye at seven months and the other at eleven months to retinoblastoma, a rare form of cancer. Despite or perhaps because of him becoming blind—we really don't know—at age three the first revelation of his musical genius became apparent when his dad, Bud, gave him a little Hawaiian style guitar. In uncharacteristic fashion—which remained a Jeff Healey attribute his whole life—he attacked playing the guitar, and within weeks the three-year-old had switched from his father's conventional way of holding it to the keyboard placement for which he became famous. Bud recollects the budding protege. "His musical skills were innate, his curiosity inexhaustible, his career path inescapable, his memory photographic, and his brain like a computer."

Jeff's first love was neither rock nor jazz but country music, and he loved Johnny Cash most of all. When Johnny Cash albums came out, Jeff learned them immediately. He decided to move on from country once he figured out that he could play just about any song with three chords. It must be a first in music—with the possible exception of Mozart—for a child to find a whole genre of music too easy to hold his interest.

When Jeff was eight, he got the chance to meet his idol but was too tongue-tied to ask Johnny any of the questions he had been planning for weeks to ask. And now, there he was at the building entrance, not tongue-tied but certainty uncertain of what to do, and no one waiting to answer any questions. I desperately motioned to a few student government people as to where Jeff stood, imploring a delegation to spring into action. Still, no one moved. It was not so much reluctance as a collective deer-in-the-highlights scenario that had the students spellbound. Not knowing that anything is supposed to happen will do that.

So, I greeted the great Jeff Healey and his parents like a dolt, looking around as I made small talk, trying to figure out how to hide the fact that he was a complete surprise to me and everyone else but fooling no one. His auditory acuity probably picked up my bewilderment and fakery as soon as I opened my mouth. The fact that the president of the university saw what I saw and motioned to me as I motioned to the students didn't help. He just assumed that the Jeff Healey handling was my failure, which I never did try to correct. An explanation that student government people only work with us to the extent that we do not try to run their operation would likely have been lost to his view of the world.

For all the confusion, Jeff Healey didn't seem to mind, or least he had too much class to let on. What I remember most about our exchange as the ragged Jeff Healey Award for Students with Disabilities was launched was how bloody humble he was. He was also very decent, modest, and shy in the glow of a limelight he could not see and—while not playing music—may have concluded he didn't deserve. I thought, doesn't this guy know that rock stars are supposed to be loud and self-centred and create havoc? But Jeff Healey was never going to be accused of being conventional.

The whole event was uneventful. Uneventful words were punctuated by gaps of silence in the absence of music. Beyond acknowledging that he was in attendance, there was no mention of Jeff's astonishing achievements of very recent years. We had the great Jeff Healey in our presence, with permission to use his name, and no one thought about playing his music. No one considered that playing recorded music from the Jeff Healey Band might showcase how bloody far a student with a disability can go with a bit of support. And with Jeff Healey actually agreeing to attend the event, it never occurred to the mystery person who invited him that he might further agree to provide live music, which would have rocked the house and had media people putting the Jeff Healey Award on the map. No one put a fraction of the effort that that three-year-old put into playing his new guitar on his lap, so he could attack both the instrument and his future life, into having Jeff Healey in attendance.

As a young blind child with an innate drive, Jeff had lots of time and little distraction. (What might be the cumulative effect of Netflix and the like on young people's drive, hunger, and willingness to put in the time required to achieve mastery? How do the many sophisticated distractions today—to which I too am addicted—erode accomplishment to the point where we are no longer even capable of knowing what we are missing? Not knowing that we are missing something does not mean we don't miss it; it simply contributes to the nihilistic angst that we feel but cannot articulate. What meaning can anyone extract from being solely a consumer of entertainment? If we consume but never articulate, who are we? Serious questions.)

Musical prowess always starts with listening to music, however original we think we are. And if country music lost its lustre because it was too easy, his next love, jazz, does not suffer from being simple. Its inherent discordance and infinite variations might best be described as complex. While he played, recorded, and became famous for rock and blues, he amassed a rare and unique collection of over 30,000 78 rpm records, with particular interest in the impossible-to-find jazz records from the 1920s and '30s. Impossible, that is, for a sighted person, but not apparently for Jeff Healey. (This follows upon my observed phenomenon of the banality of self-evident truths; though seemingly common, they are often impossible, if not for the fact that they are in evidence right before our eyes.)

In 1990, Jeff hosted a radio show on CIUT at the University of Toronto, and later he had a show called *My Kind of Jazz* on CBC. Both shows not only highlighted Jeff Healey's distinctive deep voice and encyclopedic knowledge of what most people might call obscure jazz but, of necessity, featured selections from his unique personal musical collection. The show was hugely popular, and listeners had to conclude that this voice was quite different from what they had assumed they knew of the blues rocker as a performer. Jeff Healey's range of articulation was wide, deep, multidimensional, complex. And perhaps other worldly.

So how did Jeff Healey do it? How do people without sight do it? How did all my students over the years do it? How do any of us do it? How do we survive, how are some people able to elevate *survive* into *thrive*? If life's purpose is to seek and luxuriate in material-world advantage, how is there purpose in living without or with less than what it is that the world has to offer?

Perhaps the modern, very modern, view that purpose derives from external sources is flawed. Perhaps the less modern extant view that purpose is determined by internal interpretation of the world is a beginning. Because the modern external view will always let you down. Hardship and loss always come, with uncertainty lurking close by. And knowing this, accepting this, and not confusing meaning with happiness might begin to lend itself towards insight and resilience:

> People have an unbelievable capacity to face and overcome things they don't understand, and not only that, that's essentially what gives life its meaning ... Every time you're exposed to a part of the world that you don't understand you have the possibility of rebuilding the structures that you use to interpret the world.[7]

---

7. Jordan Peterson, "Reality and Sacred Lecture," in Jim Proser, *Savage Messiah: How Dr. Jordan Peterson Is Saving Western Civilization* (New York: St. Martin's Press, 2019), 183.

The possibility of a Phoenix-like recovery in response to hardship is far more optimistic than a nihilistic avoidance of pain. Out of grievance, indifference, or lack of curiosity people are increasingly embracing a trendy nihilistic means of coping. I observe bemused, occasionally amused (since I am not nihilistic), and wonder, How do people spring out of bed in the morning eager to engage faux purpose in shopping and surrender to appropriate abstract causes? Confronting life as it is, painful as it is, seems both more difficult and more meaningful than consuming or abstracting what life isn't.

Not everyone finds it within themselves to elevate from survive to thrive, even with every advantage. And though I don't know anything about what he did or did not believe, the ascendancy of Jeff Healey, his articulation of purpose through music, is miraculous. To those high school students throwing themselves against a locker in mock exaggeration of getting out of the way of the blind guy coming down the hallway, miraculous is hidden or denied by mockery. It questions without exaggeration who is actually blind. The self-assessed cool student probably didn't foresee that Jeff Healey was about to be regarded as the coolest guy on the planet.

I know the unseeing type; you've met him, and we have all heard his brutal unseeing proclamation, framed as a rhetorical question. Looking and fearing without knowing, he says, "How can anyone live like that?" I often make the same proclamation about material-world adherents. People pride themselves for living unencumbered lives, investing wholly in material-world certainty, without questioning purpose, origin, or where all the extraordinary aspects of a life we've privileged to receive might lead. All these decades later, I wonder if it ever occurred to the guy throwing himself against the locker that maybe he missed an opportunity, that maybe God had placed a genius on his path for a reason. Seems doubtful, but *if not for the grace of God* precedes *whomever God places on our path*, the twin pillars to our meaning in life. As such, forgiveness and the opportunity to learn something from that aborted exchange exist still. These decades later, if that student sees the prank for the pathetic cruelty it was, he can reframe who he was and, in asking for forgiveness, become closer to what he had hoped to be. Such is the power and spiritual potential of consciousness that we rarely acknowledge but would be less angst-ridden if we did.

Kids today are often told they can be anything, that their potential is unlimited. The message is supposed to be inspiring, I guess. But the reality is, kids are less and less resilient the more they are confronted with uncertainty, and what could be more uncertain than being told that anything is possible? Even young people intuit it isn't true, which leads to further unarticulated uncertainty. So, is the problem having unlimited potential or having to deal with limitations?

One of the things that modern psychology is increasingly telling us, is that without the limitation that a creature like us, with the structure of our consciousness, brings to bear on the world, there's no reality. That what reality is, is an emergent consequence of the interaction between something that's painfully limited like us and whatever the absolute is, which is something that is completely without borders. And what that implies, in a sense, is that without limitation there's no being, with limitation there's suffering. Without suffering then there's no being.[8]

To my limited thinking, there exists epiphany logic in the coupling of suffering and meaning. Life distilled to the elemental is this dance *between something that's painfully limited like us and...something that is completely without borders*. It is no coincidence that people who get to luxuriate in money, fame, or any material-world excess are more likely to describe themselves as being empty than those who overcome obstacles. This is not to glorify hardship, but it has to be acknowledged that meaning derives from the discordant jazz-like notes of imposed limits rather than the supposed harmony of access to everything. There would be no meaning to running a world record if anyone could do it, and, if possible, even the notion of *world record* would have no meaning. It is precisely in overcoming physical and psychological limits that greatness resides and spirituality beckons. Whatever our individual physical limitations, whatever cards we have been dealt, it is precisely what we do in the circumstances in which we reside that separates the miraculous from the mundane.

Was it miraculous or mundane when that three-year-old received and repositioned the gift of a guitar onto his lap and began to apply his "innate skills," "inexhaustible curiosity," and "photographic memory" to the limitations of blindness and inexperience? Even for a musical genius, most of the ten thousand hours required to carve meaning from limitation were likely unglamorous repetition. And, it has to be said, a three-year-old doesn't know about genius, potential, or stardom. Jeff channeled limitations that he chose to see as opportunity into a guitar that he held in a unique, weird way that worked for him, until it yielded to his articulation of the heart, which he subsequently laid out every night for years and still echoes in recorded music.

So powerful was his need to articulate that he managed to send us a new album almost ten years after his death. In 2016, an album of 12 lost tracks entitled *Heal My Soul* was released, which Jeff's wife Christie described as Jeff "sitting right next to me. I couldn't make it halfway through without bawling my eyes out." During the time leading up to his death, music was not foremost on the minds of his family and friends. "When Jeff passed there was a resounding echo among everyone who knew him. They just couldn't contemplate the fact that he was gone. Because it was always just the next step, the next fight, the next thing to overcome. It was shocking to everyone that he had finally succumbed." What best friend and album producer Roger Costa and Jeff's wife didn't know was that Jeff had kept and transcribed to modern format tracks recorded as the Jeff Healey Band was disbanding 20 years

8. Peterson, "Reality and Sacred Lecture," 187.

earlier. The tracks had never been released because of disagreements within the band, but when the rough mixes were discovered, Roger "was absolutely floored. I couldn't believe how good the tracks were … we absolutely had to make sure that we got this out there."[9]

Interestingly, the impending breakup of the band (1996 to '98) didn't just prevent *Heal My Soul* from being released for two decades; the limitations of that experience also fuelled Jeff's need to articulate. Costa writes that "during this period, songs were just flowing out of him. I think it's also in part because of the turmoil that he was going through and all the stress. There's countless tales of artists finding that real beauty comes out of adversity."

Dealing with adversity didn't necessarily make Jeff Healey become one of the world's greatest musicians, but it may have forced him to face down and conquer limitations, which comes close. Limitations gave music great meaning, which led to a realization of the qualities his father ascribed to his young son and, in time, allowed Jeff to be an *emergent consequence of the interaction between painfully limited and something that is completely without borders.*

"Well, I'm the guy who never learned to dance

Never even got one second glance

I could look but I could never touch."

Jeff Healey lived a short life. He learned to dance, got more than a second glance, and can look and touch to his heart's content. There are ten references to having sight in "Angel Eyes," and listening to and watching Jeff Healey in the opening stanzas to the music video, you would have to conclude that the guy who finally gets the girl, mystery as it may be, has insight. This more than any other Jeff Healey song is a revelation, with voice, words, and guitar harmonizing to create music without borders, a limitless result, a sum greater than its parts, more than its ten thousand preceding hours.

---

9. Henry Yates, "The Story of the Great 'Lost' Jeff Healey Album, Heal My Soul," in *Classical Rock*, May 4, 2008.

Chapter Five

HEARING FROM THE HUMAN HEART

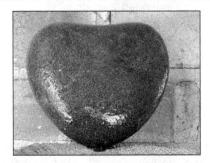

"Science may have found a cure for most evils; but it has no remedy for the worst of them all — the apathy of human beings."

Helen Keller, writer, disability rights activist (1880–1968)

I remember the film well. Patty Duke was popular in the 1960s for playing two roles as identical looking cousins on the *Patty Duke Show*. Dumb premise, since identical doesn't happen between cousins, but we liked naive in the 1960s and decided not to notice. In 1962, before double-starring in her own show, she won an Academy Award, for best actress, for her portrayal of Helen Keller. *The Miracle Worker* included Ann Bancroft, who also won an Academy Award, for best actress in a supporting role, for her portrayal of Annie Sullivan, the poor Irish worker of miracles. The script was adapted from Helen Keller's autobiography *The Story of My Life*, which recounts singular courage and resiliency against odds and circumstances that even, or especially, today are hard to believe.

When Helen was 19 months, she contracted either rubella or scarlet fever and became both blind and deaf. After years of her living in complete isolation and knowing of no other existence, her parents contemplated having her committed to an institution, which would have been a death sentence. Without the possibility of communication, without context of any kind to know herself and others, she had fits of rage, with a growing propensity for violence. Hers was a life beyond the inarticulate speech of the heart, for she barely knew what speech was.

Social isolation was not well understood at the time but in recent years has been extensively studied. The conclusion to a comprehensive contemporary literature review is as follows:

Social pain theory helps emphasize the vital role of connection with others in human behavior. Those of us living in individualistic societies are inundated with messages trumpeting autonomy and individuality. Yet, a picture is emerging that people are so vitally important to each other that social needs are ingrained in our very biology.[10]

While Helen Keller was alive and for decades afterwards, placing prisoners into solitary confinement for extended periods of time was an accepted form of punishment. In recent years, we have come to regard solitary confinement for what it is: torture. For young Helen, the isolation of sensory deprivation was further exacerbated by childhood innocence and complete incomprehension.

But just before surrendering their daughter to an institution, Helen's parents were referred to Alexander Graham Bell, who in turn recommended them to the Perkins School for the Blind. Annie Sullivan had a visual impairment and had come to Perkins because, being both illiterate and poor, it was her only chance to get an education. Annie not only became literate; she learned innovative techniques from Laura Bridgman, who was the first blind and deaf English speaker to use finger spelling and writing on hands to communicate.

Annie Sullivan was 21 and Helen Keller was 7 when they met. The film centres on their tumultuous relationship, from which grew a lifelong friendship and lives worth living. I saw the film only once in the mid to late 1960s, with my mom, and still remember the portrait of claustrophobic isolation leading to the revelation of relationship. And with the ability to articulate, to know and be known, Helen Keller embraced and transformed the world.

The child who did not know of and could not access speech became the woman who loved language, luxuriated in literature, and wrote 12 books. The child who could not be educated became proficient enough with language to go to the Cambridge School for Young Ladies before being admitted to Harvard University's Radcliffe College, where she became the first deaf-blind person to earn a BA degree. It is interesting that one of the many quotes attributed to Helen Keller is "College isn't the place to go for ideas." Perhaps because of this insight, an admirer by the name of Mark Twain introduced Helen to Standard Oil magnate Henry H. Rogers, who agreed to pay for her education. Even more impressive than succeeding and thriving at the Cambridge and Radcliffe schools is the fact that for 25 years before and after her mainstream education, Helen Keller studied to learn to speak so that others could understand her. For some passionate few, the need to give voice, articulate, and exit isolation is what matters most in life.

10. G. MacDonald and M. R. Leary, "Why Does Social Isolation Hurt? The Relationship Between Social and Physical Pain," *Psychological Bulletin* (2005): 218.

The Miracle Worker created a lot of public interest in Helen Keller's life. And with 12 books to her credit, she had certainly achieved being known. Above all else, I remember as a ten-year-old hearing about her answer to a much-asked question: Which condition is worse, blindness or deafness? That question today is fraught with political difficulty because people with disabilities do not want to have their lives described as lacking humanity or value due to their condition. A person with a disability is not a disability with a person. Still, questions like this are asked, and most respondents say blindness is worse, while only 6 percent respond that deafness is worse. But Helen Keller was never average, was always about connection, and she famously replied, "Blindness separates people from things; deafness separates people from people." The greatest connection in Helen Keller's life was with the person who served to connect her to the world. When Annie Sullivan died in 1936, Helen Keller—who had camped by her bedside for weeks—was holding her hand.

Helen Keller anticipated the central dilemma of modern life as well as the life trajectory of one of my early, most energetic students: "Many people have a wrong idea of what constitutes true happiness. It is not attained through self-gratification but through fidelity to a worthy purpose."

Tanis showed up at my door, age 15, admitted into first year university, ready to commit to her worthy purpose, and willing to tell me what I had to do to make sure she could get to do what she had to do. She was bossy, irreverent, outrageous, funny, hardworking, accomplished, one of the smartest people on the planet, and hearing impaired. She was considered difficult by most; I liked her for being refreshingly real.

Something had happened between her and her parents, and she now lived with her grandfather. She would often tell me something or some things unsolicited, and I would listen, not particularly curious, but to show I was listening I would ask an innocuous question as a logical consequence of what she had just said. More often than not she would demand to know why I had asked that question, and I would retreat to not asking questions, at which point she would ask if I was still listening. Contradiction loomed large in our relationship. Tanis demanded feedback while wanting to remain unknown. I substituted grunts of agreement for questions, and all was good.

She never did tell me how she got into university at age 15, and if she really was 15, she was the oldest, most mature 15-year-old on the planet. Whether student, staff, or faculty member, no one ever bested her in an argument, and when listening to her speak you really had to conclude that she bested the best because she was better.

She demanded more of me and more work from me than any other student. And she wasn't necessarily discreet, sensitive, or even civil. But I did notice that for all her wild advocacy and occasional histrionics, she did try to temper her more outrageous tendencies during the occasional times when I was allowed to speak.

She was my best ally in dealing with difficult emerging accommodations issues, and she could be her own worst enemy.

And I really did need her help. I had no idea how to provide services to deaf and hearing-impaired students, and she gave me the crash course that I needed. Early on the de facto response to deaf students in the post-secondary sector was to hope that they and their complex issues would go away. I was never the go-away type of person but wasn't sure how to proceed. Tanis would say, "Here's how it's done, stupid," to which I would respond, "That's a lot of information," to which she responded back, "You are slow," to which I re-responded, "Who doesn't learn complex stuff slowly?" to which she, who always demanded the last word, said, "Me."

She was right, was usually right, though she would say "always." Deferring to her brilliance was not difficult, and as the years passed, her guidance in navigating the politics around services for deaf students continued to be invaluable. Deaf students needed interpreter services, which was expensive and complicated, with interpreters in high demand and with some assignments requiring booking and paying for two interpreters. Add up class time and preparation time, then factor in the number of classes per course times the number of courses taken, and the challenge of providing interpreters becomes evident.

And then there were hearing-impaired students who did not need interpreters because they communicated by reading lips and practising speech, both skills taking years of training. The deaf community tended to be split, and the issue was politically charged according to which group one belonged to. It is easier to provide far more limited services to students who do not need interpreters, and it is also true that those who lip-read function independently in the hearing world.

Deaf students requiring interpreters are less independent in the hearing world, but they argue that sign language is their native language and should not be compromised by cost and institutional convenience. If ever I was confronted by an issue that did not have an easy answer, this was it. Tanis attacked issues—and not infrequently people too—pushing, aggressively advocating, but never beyond the reach of what was possible. That is, she recognized student rights, she acknowledged what I was up against, she did not put herself on a pedestal or virtue signal, and together we did what we could without compromise, while remaining in the realm of real. She wasn't radical so much as radically persistent.

During her first year at university she considered me to be on probation. She never said as much, but not being a shrinking violet, Tanis's views were well-known. Once my probation expired, she decided I was all right and, that being the case, we should change the world, practically speaking of course. I never saw myself changing the world, though I could envision Tanis's bull-in-a-china-shop approach to life as either getting us into deep trouble or changing everything, so I agreed. We wrote and published a disability guide, we wrote a research paper for government, and then when the provincial ministry changed their post-secondary funding for students with disabilities, we helped organize students into a national association, which still exits. And that was just the start. We were opposites, but we shared a work ethic that did not allow for saying without doing, a quality I still value above all others. Tanis's take-no-prisoners approach to life was greeted with mixed results by other students. Many students were intimidated by and critical of her; others admired her right up until they came against her righteous wrath. Still, everyone had to admit, if Tanis said it, she did it.

Her assertiveness rubbed off on Scott. He was shy, quiet, and did what he was told—that is, what Tanis told him to do. Still, he had his own ideas, and he came in to see me one day with a question. Scott was profoundly hearing impaired, and despite being shy he was very proficient in his ability to communicate. This was way back at the beginning of time, 1984, and Scott had read that our prime minister, Pierre Elliot Trudeau, had announced his intention to retire from office. Scott admired the prime minister and asked if I knew of any events the PM was speaking at that he could attend. I responded, "Just give me a minute."

I motioned for Scott to sit down, which I knew he would not do, both shyness and the inhospitable nature of my office/corridor being compelling reasons. I got the phone number for the prime minister's office from the operator, called it, and explained to a bewildered but patient functionary that I had a few admirers who would love to meet the prime minister before he drove away in his Mercedes. I was briefly put on hold, and when the functionary returned, I was offered a time and a date after question period in the House of Commons, the next day or perhaps a couple days away. I mouthed the offer to Scott, who being adept at lip-reading understood me perfectly, and he enthusiastically agreed.

It was that easy, and represents a world of easy that has completely disappeared. You could not simply call the PMO today, deal with one person, and have an appointment to meet the prime minister. You would have to be someone who has special access to a key functionary among many who would further vet your specialness for political advantage, which, if it existed, might result in a distant meeting at a controlled event for a very limited time.

Today security alone would deter most people from attending the House of Commons during question period. I don't know why we indiscreetly skipped question period, but I do remember that we simply walked into the House of Commons and stood at the spot that had been described to me, where the prime minister presumably would show up and meet our little band. We probably didn't want to risk getting stuck upstairs in the gallery and possibly miss the prime minister, who was known to vacate quickly and move more quickly.

There were four of us, Tanis included. In principle, she wasn't interested in joining, for reasons I didn't ask for, but when I pressed her for a conclusive answer before I extended the invitation to someone else, she agreed to come. Which I knew she would. I thought it might get interesting if the prime minister asked Tanis a question or if Tanis took it upon herself to lecture him about what he could and should be doing to help students with disabilities. I thought about suggesting discretion but realized that if Tanis did rail against injustice the prime minister would recognize her brilliance and just as likely hire her into the PMO as be offended. Besides, if I haven't made it clear yet, Tanis was her own substantial person.

Question period ended, the doors to the Commons opened, and the prime minister bounded out. Without needing prompting or direction (chances are he'd done this before), Mr. Trudeau came directly toward us, with political aides following in his wake, as the members of our little band began to quake. Which was misplaced, because the whole experience was relaxing. He called me by my first name as if we were old pals, we shook hands, and as I faded backwards, Mr. Trudeau greeted each student personally. Even Tanis was suitably charmed, but it was Scott who was given the most attention. Scott loved to canoe and had brought a copy of Bill Mason's *The Path of the Paddle* for the prime minister to sign since the PM just happened to have written the introduction. Mr. Trudeau was quite taken by this; the two became instant best friends and then proceeded to flip through the book together, admiring details in their private little world. Interestingly, the prime minister took real time, which he obviously didn't have since his aides pestered him about other pressing appointments. His non-response echoed in the great open space, their ignored repeated enticements serving to question their very existence. The image of a rhinoceros swinging his tail to keep flies from his a*s comes to mind, the many scurrying aides being the many buzzing flies.

A couple of years later, Scott came by my office to tell me that he was about to graduate. We reminisced a bit and I kidded about being abandoned by yet another student (realizing that to a minor degree I really didn't want them to leave me) and watched as Scott prepared to say something. He said that meeting with Mr. Trudeau changed his life, those being the last words we ever exchanged. I recently found out that, after graduation, Scott became a successful lawyer. *Good for you*, I thought; *guess you weren't kidding about the impact of that meeting*. I wonder if he still gets out for a carefree paddle once in a while.

Tanis's expansive intellect resulted in a compressed timeframe for her education, for realizing her many achievements, for life. In less time than should have been possible, she graduated and, while still a teenager, began a graduate program in social work. That too was soon dispensed with, and in two shakes of a dead lamb's tail, she left us to start a PhD program on the west coast.

I decided to write this book when I thought about how many students I knew intensely well during an intense time in their life, but with me not being of their life, they were soon gone. That process from intensity to nothing (bearing in mind that the ability to track through Google did not always exist) was always both bewildering and exactly how it was meant to be. Still, Tanis surprised me and made an effort to keep in touch despite the big life she had embraced and the fact that our lives were now like two ships passing in the night.

Our connection was never about our exteriors or membership in a particular tribe. On the surface—if we thought in those terms—our tribes didn't necessarily talk much. She was a deaf woman and casually mentioned one day that she was a lesbian, to which I responded, "Makes sense," and I was to later learn that she was also a Métis (Ojibwa/French Canadian); whereas I was a white heterosexual male so had no status in the ID world, which she often reminded me of and was occasionally protective of if she thought I might be faulted for not having the appropriate attributes. Bottom line: What I was didn't interest her much; what I did interested her a lot. I never talked of and she never asked about my wife and children. Personal stuff was not so much a no-go zone as it was irrelevant to goals, strategies, and assessing how plans in play were working out.

I was thinking about Tanis from the distant past while listening to a speaker in the effervescent present at a conference in Boston on post-secondary education and disability. The speaker was billed as something of a phenomenon, being an accomplished deaf-blind woman refugee of colour. The trajectory of Haben Girma's life is spectacularly unlikely.

I'm the first Deafblind student at Harvard Law School. Harvard excluded many groups throughout its history. When Helen Keller was applying for college, Harvard wouldn't admit her. Back in those days, Harvard only ad-mitted men. Helen's disability didn't hold her back, nor did her gender: it was the community at Harvard that chose to create barriers for women. Harvard's sister school, Radcliffe College, offered Helen Keller admission, and she received her degree in 1904.[11]

But for all her reasons to seek cover in the intersectionality of her many challenges, Haben understands what Victor Frankl learned: "the last of the human freedoms—to choose one's attitude in any given set of circumstances, to choose one's own way."

I'm in the confounding position of being both ultra-visible and invisible. People will stare—it's human nature. Eyes are drawn to people who stand out, like a black woman with a dog and strange computer in the middle of a Harvard Law School reception. People will judge—that's human nature, too. A lot of people will decide to avoid me, assuming I don't have anything of value to contribute. I can't control their actions, but I can control the message I send.[12]

I've sat through many keynote speeches from speakers with less claim to discrimination who have pontificated about the history of opposition without taking responsibility for how to roll up our collective sleeves and solve the problem. At Harvard, Haben engaged people to work with her towards finding solutions, recognizing that trailblazers can create new challenges. "The school doesn't know

11. Haben Girma, *Haben: The Deafblind Woman Who Conquered Harvard Law* (New York, Grand Central Publishing, 2020), 224.
12. Haben, *Haben*, 210.

exactly which accommodations I need. Neither do I—doing law school Deafblind is new to me, too. We engage in an interactive process. We try different strategies, one after another, until we find the right solutions."[13] Which is how Tanis and I approached problems, which is why our particular identity was not important, unless we are talking about that other identity, which we are not born into but earn over time based on what we do, called character.

Tanis was a character with character, I thought while listening to Haben, who was compelling for her sense of adventure, sense of humour, and the way she engaged people to see past her disability and communicate with her. Haben communicates with a BrailleNote computer that raises metal pins to her touch, so it acts as a tactical screen. Haben helped develop her BrailleNote to function with a Bluetooth keyboard, so that people can easily communicate with her, which BrailleNote has now incorporated into its capabilities.

Tanis never encountered a barrier that she didn't have ideas about how to solve. She was an activist in search of an outcome, and her tribe included a coalition of the willing to work. Despite her many accomplishments, all achieved in record time, she worked hard, never opting for easy in life. And she could never understand those who opted for easy. She just assumed that everyone is motivated by passions, deeply held opinions, and the need to act. She didn't suffer fools, the symbol of court jester to Tanis being the apathetic fool.

For months or even years I wouldn't know anything about her, and then Tanis would appear at my door as if we had planned to meet and discuss plans for conquering the next major problem. One day she mentioned that she had adopted a deaf girl from Jamaica, this while being single, scattered by graduate school, having piecemeal employment and always projects in progress, and living in a city without family or potential caregivers. It was an impossible undertaking, which I knew she'd find a way to do well.

A couple years pass, maybe a few more—it was always hard to keep track. Tanis appears, always unannounced, always knowing she'd be welcomed, and this time in a wheelchair. She wasn't sure what the cause was but dispassionately speculated it was likely something neurological for which the recovery possibilities were poor. Still, she assured me, the big ball of wax called her life would be fine. And it was, until she died soon after, age 37.

My mantra in these increasingly ideological times, and, especially on a university campus, where much remains theoretical, is to keep it real. For all her potential claim to intersectionality, Tanis was an exemplar of keeping it real towards getting it done. Our relationship may seem strange as described in consideration of these identity-obsessed political times. But we worked well together, always, and shared a natural like-minded collegial bond. Ideological outrage is no substitute for hard-won outcome. Profound insight can come in seemingly trivial, innocuous packages.

---

13. Haben, *Haben*, 224.

The life we have been loaned is either about nothing or everything, and if everything, we need to examine the contents of the innocuous for existence of the incredible. Maybe in addition to *whomever* God places in our path, our purpose lies in *whatever* problem God places in our path. Grinding through work with calloused hands and fatigue that burns not only might alleviate a problem but might just be the solution.

Chapter Six

INARTICULATE SIGHT OF THE HEART

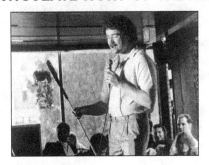

*"The eye with which I see God is the same eye
with which God sees me."*
**Meister Eckhart, German theologian, Dominican mystic preacher
(1260–1328)**

Thirty some years on and I'm supposed to be immune to surprise. Experienced professionals on career paths pride themselves on having seen it all, which has the potential for their claim of professionalism to mask wilful blindness. Immunity from surprise is to forgo wonder, so it's maybe best to be an inquisitive lifelong amateur.

It is our daily dilemma. Bookended between workday drudgery and the freight train of distraction, we sleepwalk through life, seeing only the well-trodden path, thinking we can see what there is to see. Ours is not the blindness of darkness but the sightless "light-filled milky sea" contagion of Jose Saramago's novel *Blindness*.

This was my unprofessional thought as I recently broke through the hubris of habit and saw three blind women walking close together through the corridors of the university. Three huddling shufflers came to a wide-open section of a student gathering space. Passing students were engaged by groups of students who hawked membership to a club or, if willing to subvert critical thinking for borrowed meaning, were furiously recruited to join an ideological cause. For all the edginess of essential faux causes, these practitioners of unoriginal make university campuses the epitome of conventional. A place where unseeing is required.

Except for those unseeing and unseen. They were slow, challenging my habitual need to move quickly. Had I not slowed, I would have suffered my own "light-filled milky sea" sightless contagion. Alice was a familiar face and the oldest, say 40, and the other two women, about half her age, were new to the campus, the three a veritable wayfaring team, each a tactical point of reference for the other but none in command of direction. Moving in tandem slowness and occupying a wide berth, they managed to frustrate hurrying students without being noticed. They were a spectacle to be avoided but not seen—the spectacular shooting star that streaks across the sky as we watch a Netflix original huddled together inside.

Alice, who had negotiated these paths for some years, was actually the most anxious of the three. She seemed to have an idea in her head that did not correspond to the reality of their barrier-fraught route. The two younger women did not seem anxious so much as resigned to being lost. I could not determine if their resignation was to the present moment or to where their lives might lead. Curiously, none of the women had a guide dog.

Braking from slow to shuffling inertia, I waited suspended between offering help and continuing on. They had just made a guess and veered right but, guessing wrong, ended up in dead space, surrounded by objects, regrettably garbage bins, without the possibility of moving forward. I approached silently but did not speak; they backed up, corrected, and continued to feel their way towards a destination. Their way-finding was cumbersome, awkward, the product of trial and error. Several times they seemed to be in real trouble but then recovered before I could offer help. And that is their daily dilemma.

They have to make their own way in this world, and while most of us think about offering help, we usually don't. We justify it with the aforementioned *they have to make their own way in this world,* but we are reluctant to admit that what they do on a daily basis exists on the threshold of impossibility. The truth, which I conveniently neglected in that moment, is that the offer of help is rarely the wrong call. Even when help is not needed, a heartfelt offer is usually gratefully received for the human connection that it is. Still, we hesitate and then don't. The isolation between humans is mostly self-imposed.

The three continued into the large student run café, with a chaotic menagerie of students sitting at or scrambling for tables, a long lineup of students waiting to order food from the busiest food service on campus, and a backed-up crowd of students waiting to pick up their ordered food in front of the grill. Suffice to say, it is a complicated place requiring high visual acuity in order for anyone to function. Out-maneuvering students waiting for infrequently available tables requires stealth, assertiveness, and sight. Those not jumping at the first hint of movement at an occupied table are destined to forever stand. And then there is the mosh pit where students gather to receive the food they have ordered, this being the lowest and most intense form of lunchtime hell.

I followed. I was very familiar with this place, mixing it up with the vultures on a daily basis to get my bagelwich fix. I watched, again suspended, wanting the women to be marvels of resourcefulness and assertiveness. I wanted the crowd to swarm with kindness and consideration whenever resourcefulness and assertiveness flagged. But no, the women remained unseen, even or especially when contact was made. Still, they muddled through the line under Alice's determined lead.

The two twenty-year-olds were inclined to wait whenever the little group got stuck, but Alice had done this before, her whole life actually, and was not deterred by mere obstacles. The younger women looked as if they would do anything to be spared the logistical necessity of asking for help. They wanted to fit in inconspicuously — worlds apart from being invisible — and asking for help was sticking out. I know that look on the faces of twenty-year-olds — three daughters will do that — wanting to stay cool while standing on metaphoric tracks with a train bearing down hard.

Alice was a good influence on the younger women, having stopped caring long ago about appearance and the cool factor. She was courageous and not limited by trendiness. She managed to secure a table and recruited someone to keep it for them until, or if ever, they got through the lineup for food. The twenty-year-olds stood together lightly touching, not wanting the chain broken, their tether to something familiar. Curiously, each had a fashionable blonde streak in her hair, a flair for fashion, sight unseen. God love them, I was glad they cared about how they looked, had someone who cared about how they looked.

Waiting to get their food in the pit after paying was difficult, constantly bumping into people who gave dirty looks they felt but could not see, their only spoken word during the entire ordeal a heartfelt, very Canadian "Sorry." None of the three responded when their number was called. The girls at the cash had explained that they needed to keep their receipt with a number on it to be able to match it to their order when it was ready. She did not consider that the girls could not see the number on the receipt, and yet each clung to her receipt as if a tight grip might save the day. This was the point where I would have to intervene — but no, Alice took charge once again with raised voice, and ready food was matched to tightly held receipt. Crisis averted; lunch is served. Such is the trajectory of some lives.

Thirty years and thousands of students later and I can't give you meaningful insight into the beauty and complexity of these women's lives. I left once they sat down. I was curious, but it did not feel right to remain observing the next challenge of the next minute, or the one after that, without end. They began talking and eating, comfortable together, so not all about barriers. Their lives have much more to offer than barriers for those willing to see, perhaps from stylish blonde streaks to knowledge about the meaning of life.

I've always thought this about my students: how in the world will they make their way in this life? The intensity of my question has only increased with age. The conventional wisdom is that twenty-year-olds will learn from the chaos of that day, every day, and they will change and find a way to cope. People do. And of course, it is true. I just don't understand how. Wonder and admiration may add up to awe but doesn't necessarily provide insight.

Maybe I am simply perplexed because I want to believe that there is more that this life has to offer, the surface struggle belying something profound and worthy. Understanding is not way-finding. Much of life is interpretation, but there is also the objective fact that some people have cards stacked spectacularly against them. Coping does not explain, may explain away. Do our lives mean—is our daily grind no more than—coping with difficulties or luxuriating in petty comforts? Or does blindness allow more for seeing less—that is, deeper feeling, even if more painful; more insight, even if for what has been denied? Is depth of character a blessing or a curse if viewed through the lens of loss? And then there is this elemental question in the spirit of *the first shall be last and last shall be first:* will those who cope with, see through, blindness be first to have their eyes opened to the inarticulate speech of our archetypal yearning heart?

• • •

My dearly departed mother loved Gord Hope for the simple fact that he was a good Catholic boy. He wasn't a fallen Catholic; he wasn't someone who paid lip service to Catholic teachings; he was the real deal as a practitioner, and as a human being. Seems simple enough, but it is increasingly a rare phenomenon. The same for adherents to other religions. And, most regrettably, the same for people who continue to live according to standards, a code, common values, and ways of life outside of self.

Mom was accepting of almost everything, except she could never quite understand how people could refuse to go to church, how they could not understand that the Catholic Church was the perfect model for how to live life well, both virtuously and practically. In this sense, Gord made perfect sense to her; her seven fallen children, not so much. Still, Mom never withheld for what she did not understand.

When I met Gord, he was in the middle of completing a PhD. I'd like to say I helped him in some tangible way, but it isn't true. More than even the most accomplished of the pioneers with disabilities of the 1980s, he was resourceful and resilient to the core. I can hear my mom attributing this to being a good Catholic and drawing upon the grace of the Holy Spirit. I can feel my skepticism of the time, and shame in the present. She was right about just about everything we doubted, so why question her about what she felt deepest?

Gord may be the only person on earth who moved faster, more frantically, and with greater purpose than me. I never saw him stumble, seem lost, or bump into anything, and I wonder if it ever occurred to him that a reed-thin white cane is a poor defence against the world. In all things, he seemed utterly fearless.

The general public tends to regard obtaining a PhD as proof of intellectual superiority. But the process is bloody grind more than brilliant mind. The three Rs of reading, writing, and research all require excellent vision. Doing a degree at any level is obviously much tougher for blind than for sighted students, requiring far more time, perseverance, and the patience of a saint. In the 1980s, I would say it was impossible for a blind person to complete a university degree if not for that fact that Gord and a very few others did just that. Completing a PhD is on a whole other level of impossibility that Gord managed to make possible.

Services for blind students were very limited then. Reading technology was in its infancy. For example, Kurzweil reading machines—then advanced technology— were primitive, irritatingly monotone, highly inaccurate, about the size of a refrigerator for an exorbitant cost, and mostly unavailable even if a student wanted access to one. Braille was dependable, but it took months to receive an ordered book, which was awkward to use, a single print book being several encyclopedia-size volumes. Needless to say, spontaneous reading for pleasure or for research was not an option. Books recorded on tape increasingly became an option but were also cumbersome, taking some months to obtain, even when professors were willing to give us their reading lists early. So simple, but on this point at this time the faculty response was, as the saying goes, like herding cats. Volunteers were the best resource, with some people volunteering hundreds of hours of drudgery, which was essential but without any recognition.

Gord didn't only persevere, which would have been remarkable enough; he sloughed through his life of many vicissitudes with an ain't-life-grand attitude, at all times. (Reminds me of a *The Far Side* cartoon where a young guy in hell is happily working away, pushing a wheelbarrow and whistling. Two devils are watching, and one says to the other, "You know, we're just not reaching that guy.") Gord exuded happiness not only with sincerity but with complete conviction. In his presence, you just knew you were in the vortex of a consciousness that chose to be happy. You just knew.

I can't do Gord's happiness with every advantage in the world, and he did it, always, without a hint of insincerity. He was a smart guy, so it was not that he was unaware of what he was missing. But it is precisely in the perception of what we miss that scarcity resides. It is not from the small speck of our existence that perspective is determined but from the expansiveness of consciousness alive with possibility and wonder. Gord did happy, gratitude, and impossible by virtue of what he envisioned rather than what was missing; then he graduated for the third time and was gone.

It used to amuse us sibs that Mom would skip the news and sports for her perusal of the obituary section from our daily paper. It was what old people did who were losing their grip on this world and fearing what might follow. We were wrong. Her life was ever present and vibrant, and, most noteworthy, devoid of fear, especially fear of death. She always knew what would follow, which amused us, being young and stupid as we were. That death thing was so depressing, even if we bothered to give it any life by attempting to think of it as other than a distant abstraction. Why sweat the obits for people you hardly knew? (As I finished the last sentence, I realized that I may be writing this book as penance for not sweating the obits when I was young and, of course, not listening to my mother at all times…)

Then as now we have to learn first what death isn't, before we can begin to learn what death is. And death isn't distant or an abstraction or only happening to everyone else. Most of all, death isn't the *other*, the one we will never meet, which leads to a beginning of understanding about what death is: even as we live, death lurks as a certainty, so its denial negates an aspect of self. The 90-year glimpse between birth and death is our moment of either stupidity or revelation. I like to think of long life as a glimpse, a burst, a historical heartbeat bookended by transformation and awakening. Given the reality of death and the unreality of modern materialism, much of life's purpose may be about listening, seeing, examining, and finding perspective. The obits are our reminder to us, of us, of the need to forsake stupidity for revelation, including the reality of death, and given that death lasts a whole lot longer than life, it may have more significance.

I now peruse the obits every day, and from somewhere beyond, my mother approves that I have forsaken youth and stupidity—well, at least youth. It isn't just that I read the obits. Over the years what I have extracted from reading has evolved. For reasons I don't fully understand, I don't want to miss people's passing, whether or not I knew them. I suspect that obits are commonly read with a sense of schadenfreude—that is, to secretly delight in another's misfortune as a means of assuaging our lonely slice of fear. But of course, that reaction will soon bite you in the bum, as another's misfortune is our misfortune. Turns out John Donne was right: "No man is an island, entire of itself; every man is a piece of the continent." We are in this together, whether we like the concept or not. Revelation can be as simple as acknowledging the obvious.

My parents' good friends, the ones I silently watched from our kitchen table those decades ago, populated the obits until they were no more. They and endless other strangers, still of us though not among us, a life distilled into three trite and poignant paragraphs. Or many whose lives ended far too early after a courageous (courageous, being always true, is not a cliché) battle with cancer. The most heartbreaking—the death of children, young people, sudden accidents—the most likely to be framed in cliché, though no less true for the awkward expression—and though written by a stranger, read by strangers, it is to us about one of us, no separation between us, though we pretend not to know, but somehow my mother did, as we all will soon enough.

Gord's obituary in the *Ottawa Citizen*, February 24, 2016, four days after he died, age 62, began "A man with a heart larger than life," equal parts predictable cliché and searing insight. Still, in the modern material world, a heart cannot be larger than life; in fact, it cannot be anything other than a physical organ, of predictable size, efficient at pumping blood, though completely without intention. In the new paradigm, notions of the heart as more than this are barely tolerated even as a symbol. A heart beats a finite number of times and then stops, which we call death, cells that lived and are no more. Many, maybe most, people fight for this narrative, and there is palpable resistance to that other archaic notion of life beyond the obits, a reality beyond the physical world.

Problem is, the widely accepted modern explanation of death isn't just unsatisfying—it isn't true. There are reasons in science, in logic, and the self-evidence of consciousness that speak to more, a more beyond our wildest imagination. We cannot summarize 90 years of a person's essential being or capture their inarticulate speech in three paragraphs. We can only hint at the inarticulate grieving of those left behind. We feel sadness for those who have passed, but maybe we have it backwards.

I learned much from reading little. Gord's obit said he was a very involved person; it was always going to be this way. For most people, coping with blindness is isolating. The world is a visual installation; relationships are seen more than heard. Gord's list of active involvement was staggering. He contributed to organizations like he used to walk though campus—full charge at breakneck speed. Disability organizations, accessible media organizations, organizations unassociated with disability, all of which he only stopped contributing to "when his focus had to be diverted for his own health needs." Yeah, that death thing can really cut into achieving altruistic goals.

Technology has changed the lives of persons with disabilities in recent years, especially people who are blind. Voice recognition software is accurate, inexpensive, and relatively easy to use. Gord's PhD tribulations would have been far less extreme had he been engaged in the three Rs today. Still, too often technology is regarded as the pinnacle of human development rather than as a tool for connecting humans. While assessing accessible transportation systems on a train between Ottawa and Montreal, Gord was asked about the brave new world of technology. He laughed and responded, "If I'm going to get lost, I'd rather get lost with someone."

It is for his many and varied relationships with people that Gord Hope is most remembered. I learned that Gord and I have in common that we each have three daughters. "He would have been a great dad," I can say with conviction, even without having seen him for 30 years. Seems silly to say, but anyone who ever met Gord would agree.

Like, for example, Pope John Paul II. Gord was chosen to read the first Scripture at the papal Mass in Ottawa in 1984. (I happened to have lived across the street from the field where approximately one million people gathered for this historic occasion, but I didn't go. Guess I thought I'd go the next time J.P. was in town. There really is no accounting for youth.) After the reading, Gord received an unscripted, unexpected personal blessing from the pope, who was obviously personally moved. Pope John Paul II and Gord Hope were very likely the two people my mother most admired while she was alive, though don't tell her seven children.

I only learned about Gord's papal blessing from reading online posted messages that the funeral home had set up. I immediately wished I could tell my uber Catholic mother but realized that she was at the papal mass and must have known. I don't remember her ever telling me about the blessing, which was odd since she was aware that I worked with Gord and it was probably one of the highlights of her life. Although we talked often, I was not part of, was resistant to, her Catholic world, and perhaps she just didn't tell me. Worse, she probably did and I wasn't listening. A heart can articulate, but that doesn't mean it will be heard. A silver lining to this truism is that the unheard heart is patient, bides its time, and full hearing is restored decades later. The dormancy of heartfelt wisdom.

I was thinking about my mother reading the obit comments about Gord and came across this entry: "We shared many good times and walked him around the grounds where Pope John Paul II celebrated mass." Signed Bernie and Shirley Hurley. They were close friends of my parents and neighbours, living two doors down from us when we were young. They shared mom's Catholic vision of life, this one and the next. Mom would have smiled in defiance to modern world assumptions about the arbitrariness of connection.

• • •

This story happens to have a second larger than life figure who shaped my views about the purpose of being and nature of experience, who also happens to have been blind and named Gord. Gord Paynter was a self-proclaimed and universally acknowledged inspirational comic. Given that the nature of comedy tends to hinge on irreverence, the earnestness of inspiration seems an odd bedfellow. Do you want to be funny or to impart a message? Though not having a formula for comedic success, Gord managed to rock the house with laughter and still the audience with a heartfelt, hungrily received inspirational message. Every time.

The story he told—which I heard a number of equally moving times—begins when he was informed that he might eventually go blind. He reacted as an 18-year-old, which is to say that he ignored an adult pronouncement and proceeded to throw caution to the wind. He was a diabetic but lived as if he was not. At age 22, he hitchhiked through Europe by himself, which in 1976 was what young people did as a rite of passage. The comfort and convenience of all-inclusive faux-travel had not yet displaced true, if occasionally challenging, adventure. Between being told that he might go blind and his European tour, he had lost some sight, but he could still see.

He describes being in a friendly neighbourhood pub in Wales one memorable evening. He remembers sitting and sipping on a good beer, a pink fuzzy fog descending onto his field of vision. Despite forewarning, Gord was not prepared, and yet in a heartbeat, he was blind. He did not know anyone; he could not tell anyone. He managed to pay and leave the pub but did not know how to get back to his hotel. He literally felt his way along a row of hedges to his hotel. He went to bed wishing the nightmare away, only to wake into the absence of pink, fog, or any light. The nightmare of dark was to be visited upon the light of day for the rest of Gord's life.

With this thought in mind, I took an unscheduled break. I was restless and wanted to walk. My defence against the world and the anxiety it causes is to move.

Movement is proof that nothing is set, a chance that bad can change, even if from bad to worse. The irony is that these dark moments may be what we have most in common as human beings, but it tends not to be where we connect. I am between sessions at a conference on mental health, and wandering off Yonge Street I am curious about the progress of the massive renovation to St. Michael's Cathedral. The church is open, it is empty, the renovation is finished. I sit briefly—always briefly, since sitting is not movement—and try to reframe. A good place to reframe, but it is not working.

The cheapness of life, the frivolity of how we live, emblematic of Yonge Street two blocks away, pervades the quiet and stillness of where I briefly sit. It amazes me how little conversation we engage in regarding why we are here and where we are going, and I want to have that conversation. This book's conversation is within the context of early death, individual hardship, and seemingly pointless loss. Which leads to a troubling question: Who am I to attempt to write about the inner working of people's experience and suffering from the outer perspective of my small world? If we are merely of the physical world, I am appropriating their voices. Still, if there is more, if this life is more than the human speck in which I presently reside, then perhaps failing to investigate meaning is misappropriating opportunity.

Maybe compassion for those who suffer is both all too human and not quite an accurate interpretation of people's lives. It is estimated that there may have been about 100 billion lives who have proceeded us on earth throughout time. And I wonder, do they look back in sympathy to those of us still living, stuck in advance of, and in fear of, death? Maybe those who suffer most do so for those attached to the faux comfort of earthly purgatory, a spiritual ennui of suffering, though we don't know it. Maybe the story of Christ—suffering, sacrifice, and resurrection—is both true and the true trajectory of our lives. Maybe the Christ within us, the one we deny, whose voice we do not appropriate but would be fulfilled if we did, is the only story of our lives. I had these thoughts sitting still, before the blur of movement again.

In conversation, Gord doesn't talk about his struggles as much as how he was saved by comedy. As a kid Gord loved people like Red Skelton, Bill Cosby, and George Carlin and thought, *That looks like a nice way to make a living.* This thought was more than simply an aversion to work; Gord was a natural. "I was the class clown, trying to get the teacher laughing. Later I would try my jokes on waiters, bartenders, and taxi drivers, always challenging myself to get a laugh from strangers."

After having dabbled in comedy for some years, in 1984 he performed a routine at Yuk Yuk's in Toronto to audience acclaim, and a ham was born. And being a natural ham, Gord would likely have said (he and I did participate in mutual *punishment* on a number of occasions, so I have licence to speculate), "I guess that makes me a pig." Most important, that audience acclaim got him regular ongoing comedic gigs. For a young passionate man struggling with dependency and isolation imposed by blindness, the importance of finding his own particular calling cannot be underestimated. Two years later, he met his wife, and he was on his way. No doubt the two events are related, and the order in which they occurred is likely the way it was meant to be.

Gord loved getting laughs from strangers, and the desire for validation through comedy can never be fully satisfied. All serious comics have this serious affliction. They seem so casual, so relaxed, but tend to agonize over how to differentiate their act from all the other validation-addicted comics out there. But Gord had a unique story to tell and decided to combine laughter and tears, with a potent result.

It was early in Gord's inspirational comedy combo routine that I had the privilege of catching the act and meeting Gord. That meeting resulted in Gord being booked at our university for several memorable performances. Watching Gord—never quite the same routine and always highly interactive with an audience he could not see— one could not help but see that his heartfelt humour and personal story comprised the inarticulate speech of his irreverent wounded heart.

Embracing humour acted as therapy for Gord after he became blind. Gord's humour and story have much to do with blindness, but Gord's extroverted act made people understand that blindness—and by extension any disability—should not be confused with who a person is. The worst aspect of disability is not the condition but the extent to which it isolates, and Gord was never going to feel as he did while feeling his way along a row of hedges to his room from that pub in Wales.

Standing in front of an audience he didn't know and likely would never encounter again, Gord's skilled delivery and personal warmth was all about connection. The story of Gord becoming blind is frightening, but he managed to make people feel comfortable, laughing with and not at Gord's predicaments. Exiting tragedy, Gord told the audience he liked to BBQ, which may seem unusual for someone who is blind. He admitted it could be challenging, since, as inevitably happens, "wayward weenies wander off the grill." He continued, "You're familiar with the five second rule. They've expanded that window of rescue for blind barbecues to ten minutes."

One night he took an evening off to try Brantford's new casino. "I thought I'd try the slots. Boy, was I upset when I found out I'd just lost $300 to a payphone." Hoping for a miracle, Gord said that a naturopath put him on a diet of 50 carrots a day.

Gord claimed to be an exemplar of marriage. He said he and his wife never lost their temper. "We fight, but she never yells. All she does is move the furniture."

My favourite Gord Paynter joke, delivered with a thick Scottish accent, augmented by his Celtic complexion and thick, shaggy red hair, was as follows: A man wearing a tartan kilt goes up to a young lass and says, "Put yer hand up me kilt!" The young lass obediently complies before withdrawing her hand abruptly, crying, "Oh, it's gruesome!" To which the randy Scotsman says with a leer, "Put yer hand up me kilt again and see if it *grew* some more!" Editorial note: these performances were in the late 1980s into early 1990s, when people, even young people at university, still had a sense of humour. No comedian would tell such a joke on a university campus today for fear of being accused of sexually harassing a member of the audience or contributing to rape culture.

Comedians who cut their teeth performing on university campuses for peanuts such as Jerry Seinfeld would never perform on a university campus today. Humour need not be outrageous, but it is rarely funny without being somewhat subversive. Universities, the university experience, used to be about exploring subversive issues before surrender to the conventional and predictable world. With their safe spaces and narrow ideologies, universities are *the* place of strictest conformity, all in the name of tolerance, inclusion, and freedom of speech. Resulting in this question: Is the inability to see our human foibles and the irony inherent to our earnest ways a form of wilful blindness?

Gord was a self-described sports fanatic and worked sports themes into his act. He liked to name-drop, saying that both he and Wayne Gretzky were from Brantford. "They talked about him scoring 200 goals in peewee. Big deal. I was the goalie."

Gord loved basketball but indicated there was a twist for blind participants. "The winner isn't the team that gets the most points; it's the team that is able to find the gym."

When Gord tried to break into comedy in the United States, he had an interview with someone who could open doors. Unfortunately, Gord decided to begin the interview by trying to impress the someone with "I shot 6,004, the best round of golf in my life." To which the someone responded, "I don't think 6,004 is such a good score." Gord reported that he never did hear back from that someone. "Maybe I should have tried Jerry Springer. But I didn't think he'd be interested unless I'd had a hole-in-one while golfing with a naked 14-year-old."

The irony of Gord's golf joke was that he was a very good golfer, with a certified hole-in-one to his credit. He was a golf fanatic, listening to the golf channel incessantly, to his wife's frustration. He even co-hosted a call-in radio talk show on golf.

Gord's interest and appreciation of things assumed to be exclusively in the sighted world were not limited to sports. Gord, teamed up with his wife, Cath, was a world traveller who wrote extensively about travel as a columnist for *Vibrant Magazine*. Gord's column, "The Way I See It," gave a humorous and unique perspective on travel.

Gord wrote about the challenges of being a blind travel writer in a sighted world. One of my favourite examples is from his column on Istanbul, a city I have been to, noteworthy as having the worst traffic congestion in the world. It is crowded, complex, and difficult if you have sight. Without sight it is incomprehensible. Still, without bitterness and with a sense of adventure, Gord wrote about the need for him and his wife to forge their own path. "The museum of Saint Sophia was the end of our time with the tour group. We broke away. Rebels. We were fed up. Most of the tour guides we've encountered seem to be unprepared to deal with individuals with a disability. The guides appear unaware that discovering things through blind eyes takes longer. It just takes longer. Within an organized tour group, Catherine spends the bulk of her time telling me to hurry up. We're falling further and further back. We end up latching on to any tour group passing by in the hope of gleaning something about the site. That's how Catherine and I became so fluent in Japanese, Italian, and Russian."

I hadn't seen Gord Paynter for over 25 years when I learned of his death this past year. I've credited him over the years with his Scottish kilt joke, which I've subversively told many times, but, of course, not publicly because that can get you into trouble. I would have continued booking him for university performances, but the humourless campus is no place for an outrageously funny man. The extraordinary story of his life and the theme of connecting with people would be lost on a university audience obsessed by social justice causes, if an audience could even be assembled. His time has passed, and we are lesser for that heavy fact of life.

It is an odd, perhaps perverse, experience to feel loss for someone I've not thought often about for decades. Crediting Gord for his Scottish joke seems a rather thin platform for grief. Still. I recently read that our paths should have crossed at Queen's Park in Toronto in 1999, since we both received a Community Action Award from Lieutenant-Governor Hilary Weston on the same day. For some reason we did not see each other, and it occurred to me that maybe he boycotted the event once he found out that I was to be there too. In truth, I am humbled by the coincidence in consideration of the fact that in his case the award was actually deserved. More than that, he deserved a Noble Peace Prize for making people laugh and leaving them wanting more. I am among the many thousands whom Gord's departure left laughing, crying, and wanting more in perpetuity.

Chapter Seven

THE PROBLEM OF PETER

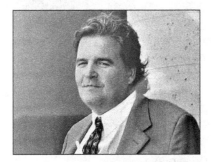

"We are slowed down sound and light waves, a walking bundle of frequencies tuned into the cosmos. We are souls dressed up in sacred biochemical garments and our bodies are the instruments through which our souls play their music."
Albert Einstein, physicist, Nobel Prize winner (1879–1955)

The Multiple Sclerosis Society's motto is "MS affects the entire family." It is a good motto, a useful reminder that there are unforeseen consequences to an individual's disabling condition. MS is an autoimmune disease whose difficulty, in addition to loss of function, is the uncertainty of worsening symptoms. Some people's symptoms plateau, and they do not lose additional function, but most cases worsen and are, ironically, called progressive. The motto is not suggesting that the disease can be shared; rather it acknowledges John Donne's famous "no man is an island" concept—that is, the consequence of one's experience is not fully one's own, however isolated he or she may feel. Family members often feel useless to help those with a disability, unaware that the best anyone can do is to help alleviate isolation. We humans exist in silos of isolation, accepting that this is what life has to offer, forgetting that acknowledging the fact of separateness may be the very thing that binds us. And hence the need to expose to the light of day what is buried deepest.

Whenever I write anything about spirituality—in other words, stray outside the purview of materialism—I feel the need to provide utilitarian balance. So this might be an appropriate moment to make a note on logic, including the noteworthy fact that logic is not exclusive to science. The greatest atheist of all time had a change of heart and reasoned that God exists, strictly in consideration of logic. For almost 50 years Anthony Flew was a devout, erudite, and prolific writer and debater, making a career out of denying the existence of God. Late in life he changed his mind, but not for reasons typical to a dramatic conversion. Flew's was no deathbed conversion, and he is unequivocal that the basis of his change of heart is about logic and not in any measure about faith. "My discovery of the Divine has been a pilgrimage of reason and not of faith."[14] Flew argues that his conversion, dramatic as it may seem, is a continuation of his lifetime commitment, with allegiance to Plato's Socratic dialogue in *The Republic*, to "follow the argument wherever it leads."[15]

Professor Dawkins's argument leads in quite another direction, and one can bet there will be no deathbed conversion or admission of doubt. The anthropic components' odds do not sway him—after all, these are only "gaps" in our understanding. The same holds when we arrive in his familiar biological playground to examine the origins of life on earth. In fact, it is under the umbrella of the highly improbable that he brings his multiverse origin theory in line with his origin of life theory—this is science, you see. And his reasoning is clever. All debates about the existence of God these days invariably invoke the award-winning end-of-argument word of not God but Darwin. Darwinism is a winner in the materialist worldview, despite being over 150 years out of date. With the odds stacked spectacularly against spontaneous assemblage of the much unproven multiverse, and with life on earth as spectacularly unlikely to just happen, both scientific events are fashioned as merely extensions of Darwinism—that is, with an infinite or at least incalculable number of universes, with an incalculable or infinite number of planets, impossible odds start to look good, likely even, and, continuing with this argument, the coming together of all anthropic components becomes inevitable.

As far as I can tell, cosmic Darwinism sort of works like this: the mindless, material universe/multiverse seeks its own creation (being unconsciously smart and highly motivated), thereby creating something, much actually, out of nothing, along with the laws that govern said material to sustain it, with the application of a sort of cosmic natural selection in order to evolve always to a higher level. Thing is—and I repeat—*it* doesn't know that it (and without intention or consciousness the totality of all things of the physical universe remains for all time a lowly non-progressing, chaotic *it*) is doing any of this. Make sense?

We humans are not divinely created; we are simply the recipients of unintended unconscious inevitability. How nice. What is not accounted for, for which a great leap still exists, is this: even with all the anthropic components in place and the universe doing its thing to make life possible on earth, there is still the unanswered question, How does life itself begin? (The question is worth asking again because it defies logic

---

14. Anthony Flew, *There Is a God: How the World's Most Notorious Atheist Changed His Mind* (New York: Harper One, 2007), 93.
15. Flew, *There Is a God*, 89.

taking for granted what science has not answered.) It might be worth considering that the composition of DNA alone has about the likelihood of just happening as all anthropic components—again, incomprehensible number, impossible odds.

Life is awesome (again, original meaning, not overused slang) every time it happens, which is to say untold trillions of times every second. Beyond the improbable odds are the breathtaking genius, ingenuity, and beauty of a fantastical system, which again, according to scientific materialism, has no awareness of its existence. To this I invoke a non-empirical articulation of the heart—the phenomenon of life, all of it, as we see, feel, and experience, is a self-evident truth of design consistent with and beyond science to explain. Natural selection contributes to an understanding but cannot account for origin, purpose, essence, or the stuff of life that is life. In a quote attributed to Albert Einstein, a dichotomous view of existence is articulated: "There are only two ways to live your life. One is as though nothing is a miracle. The other is as though everything is a miracle." Minimizing what we know to fit the nothingness of explainable scientific theories and prevalent ideological views denies life, is quite possibly death.

And who might agree with me in contradiction of Professor Dawkins? Many within the Christian church at the time of Darwin's 1859 publication of *Origin of the Species* regarded its findings as evidence of God's hand. The view that Darwin's theory of natural selection drove a spike through the heart of faith was far from an accepted fact then, though to the modern mind it is often considered proof that God is not needed. Which is very odd. During the ensuing 150 years knowledge of cell biology has expanded to a universe of complexity surrounding DNA sequencing, which renders much of contemporary notions of Darwinism, while not necessarily untrue, irrelevant. Still, the certainty of simple (natural selection explains all) over the uncertainty of complex (the more we know about DNA sequencing, the harder it is to fathom) has generalized appeal in the modern world. But perhaps we ought not to opt for simple. In Darwin's day, reverence and awe were interchangeable between science and religion in a way we moderns find difficult to comprehend, and that is too bad. Consider what Charles Darwin said of his own theory in *Autobiography*:

> [Reason tells me of the] extreme difficulty or rather impossibly of conceiving this immense and wonderful universe, including man with his capability of looking far backward and far into futurity, as the result of blind chance or necessity. When thus reflecting I feel compelled to look at a First Cause having an intelligent mind in some degree analogous to that of man's; and I deserve to be called a Theist.

Other Darwin quotes suggest agnosticism, but either way Darwin did not regard his work, in the modern sense, as disproving the existence of God. "I see no good reason why the views given in this volume should shock the religious views of anyone." If anything, Darwin reinforces my contention that science must remain dispassionate and *follow the argument wherever it leads*. "A fair result can be obtained only by fully stating and balancing the facts and arguments on both sides of each question." The earnest and dogmatic defenders of Darwinism have always been more determined and inflexible than Charles Darwin was about his own work. "If I had my life to live over again, I would have made a rule to read some poetry and listen to some music at least once every week." For all the seriousness of Darwinism and questions of origin, it is reassuring that towards the end of his life Charles acknowledged missing the opportunity to play in the sandbox, run away to the circus, exit material-world scraping for an elevating non-material-world experience or two. Survival of the uplifted.

Dawkins's arguments on the origin and evolution of life are surprisingly weak in comparison to his scientific contemporaries. Michael J. Behe's revolutionary book *Darwin's Black Box* is a must read, dissecting Dawkins's "elegantly simple" Darwinian bias and showing the "irreducible complex" nature of cellular function as evidenced in biochemistry. Behe deftly demonstrates how advances in his field have made an unquestioning adherence to materialistic Darwinism too simplistic for serious inquiry:

> In Darwin's day, the cell was thought to be so simple that first-rate scientists such as Thomas Huxley and Ernest Haeckel could seriously think that it might arise from sea mud, which would be quite congenial to Darwinism. Even just fifty years ago it was a lot easier to believe that Darwinian evolution might explain the foundation of life, because so much less was known. But as science quickly advanced and the astonishing complexity of the cell became clear, the idea of intelligent design has become more and more compelling. The conclusion of intelligent design is strengthened by each new example of elegant, complex molecular machinery or system that science discovers at the foundation of life … It is a hard fact that the scientific case for intelligent design hypothesis is getting stronger. *A separate, more dicey topic, however, concerns people's reaction to intelligent design.*[16]

Which raises a question: If, as is increasingly possible, the existence of God becomes a provable theorem (consistent with accepted scientific line of inquiry for a phenomenon that cannot be witnessed, for example, the big bang), would scientific materialists, committed atheists, and the distracted majority see what is right before their eyes? Which leads to a second question: Are we there yet?

And if not, we are left with belief in "elegantly simple" Darwinism that reduces the beauty and wonder of the world to a bland collusion of mindless brute force events. This isn't awe so much as odd and raises the question, Where exactly do we humans fit into this world, universe, multiverse? Given the materialists' framework, the question is silly; the answer, at least one that could make any sense, is not forthcoming. I suspect that materialists often catch themselves, momentarily outside their ideological captivity, and wonder at something wonderful—music, a child,

16. Michael J. Behe, *Darwin's Black Box: The Biochemical Challenge to Evolution* (New York: Free Press, 1996), 271 (emphasis added).

green—before cutting off wonder and burying reverence beneath their personal mantle of distraction and cold, calculating modernity.

In 1975, at an absurdly innocent age of 15, on the first day of his summer holidays, Peter slipped on the shore of a high Ottawa riverbank just as he began a routine unspectacular dive. Peter suffered immediate and cataclysmic damage, cleanly breaking his neck, C4–5, high up on the spinal column, at the exact same level, with the same devastating results, that Terry, his first cousin, would acquire in 1981—the year the United Nations designated International Year of Disabled Persons. So, Terry's story from my early days as an orderly was only half the story, as it affected his extended family. Peter's accident six years earlier is the reason why it did not take time for Terry to understand the enormity of his loss compared to other young bewildered men and women who become paralyzed before they have ever heard the word *quadriplegic*. Terry had steadfastly stood by his cousin's side, been one of the many people who had rallied to help Peter find a semblance of normality out of the chaos and devastation of quadriplegia. Terry had witnessed Peter struggle to cope, find equilibrium, pull a life from the embers, so he was well acquainted with the difficulty of the endless task. The conventional gestation period of some months from accident to acceptance was not Terry's experience. When he woke up, he knew. Lightning really can strike twice.

Terry had a history of falling asleep while driving and, incredibly, survived several close calls intact. He was a well-liked local lad from a well-liked local family, so the police did not make Terry face the consequences of his actions—no ticket, no warning, no suspended licence. I had not known of this link between Peter and Terry when I wrote about Terry's story. I had not intended to write about Peter until I bumped into him by pure chance. I don't believe their interwoven narratives are purely by chance. Pure chance may simply be our lack of awareness of the unseen world. Central to this concept may be the unseen hand that places people in our path. The awakening to a path may be the realization of purpose.

Forty-three years after becoming a quadriplegic, and during the Ottawa Senators' most unlikely playoff run in its franchise history, Peter posted a Facebook photo of himself in his hockey uniform, a smiling kid willing and able to take on the world. Almost immediately a friend who had been around and had known of his hockey prowess as a pre-accident teenager commented that Peter had the goods to have become a NHL calibre hockey player. Spectre of the other.

During the early weeks following his accident, it is unlikely that Peter dwelt upon the loss of his hockey career. Or maybe he survived by visualizing the freedom of effortless and unrestricted motion across a perfect clear ice surface. Maybe the solidity of frozen water assuaged his fear of drowning. Maybe he lay just below the surface, close to but not drowning, enforced breathing, connected to a hospital respirator. Time both speeded up with panic and slowed down with boredom and lack of stimulation. His world evolved around the regular mechanical noise and rhythm of the ever-present respirator. He could hear comforting voices and assurances, but it was the expression on their faces that told the truth. He was now aware of but separate from the world, from all that was familiar, from everyone he had ever known. The world into which he had fallen was completely unknown, and he did not want to know it.

Time became immobile, and Peter could count the hours between seconds. This was not the summer that was supposed to be, that made any sense, that was his to breathe into life five minutes earlier. Like most 15-year-olds before the tyranny of modern parenting, he had planned to not plan much of anything. He was going to roam and play, ferociously, savagely, always moving, never planning. Planning was for old people, cerebral and scared, sitting in chairs, and not for players and doers. But he had slipped through a portal that was not his life, and he had been conscripted to live another. The heaven of a lazy teenager summer had been exchanged for the hell of endless planning. Lying in bed having life literally breathed into him, Peter had no idea that the life that waited for him was even possible, and in 1975 neither did anyone else. Well, not exactly true, for some therapists knew that such a life as Peter was facing was possible. The question remained: Was this a life?

In 1975, Peter's survival was a phenomenon, and people reacted with a mixture of bewilderment and determination to help. Against the odds and without any sense of what those odds might be, Peter's family, especially his mother, was determined to answer the unsettled question: yes, this, Peter's life, is a life. In time, Peter would have to find a way to agree.

Pioneers who forge new paths are admired for their vision, sense of adventure, and purpose, among other qualities denoting strength. The admiration only comes after much uncertainty and adversity, if at all. Usually, forging new paths is of the pioneer's choosing. But it does happen that the most successful and determined pioneer in the world can be the most reluctant. The most reluctant are often the ones who were furthest removed from the life that they inherited: the most active, the greatest risktakers, those most drawn to adventure. In my first few weeks as an orderly, watching young men adjust to quadriplegia, I came to understand that the experience was uneven. He generally suffered most who had moved most. Those relatively few who had watched television on the sidelines of their life were less affected than those who had been terminally active. Watching television from a couch is not radically different from watching television from a wheelchair. Seems harsh, is true. And as the virtual expands, it is truer than in the recent past.

Fifteen-year-old Peter was an activity demon, a skillful player in the physical world, and was never going to forge new paths for accessibility. Complete immobility at 15 for a gifted athlete is for the butterfly to revert back to the cocoon, though if a fitting metaphor, it is not an image of comfort. Still, for some few, being a player in one domain will translate into any life lived, any cards dealt. Drive is not specific. Peter got that from his mother.

Post-accident there was that little detail about education. Peter's high school had never considered the issue of accessibility; Peter's high school principal didn't think it was possible for him to come back to the school he had attended for one short year. Stairs, washrooms—obstacles everywhere you looked—and besides, what would be the purpose of going through years of aggravation for a degree that could never be put to any use in this world? Translation: a lot of aggravation for everyone—especially the principal and his teachers—and a losing outcome for Peter. Why bother?

Peter's mother wasn't interested in why. Why is for philosophers. Peter had an education to get so that he could decide if he wanted to become a philosopher. Her approach was anything but philosophical. Without waiting for bureaucratic newspeak to cement unsettled *why* into inertia, she organized a cadre of friends and cousins, a coalition of the willing, to carry him up and down stairs, to help and feed Peter, school resources be damned. Besides, institutional resistance was never a matter of money but, rather, useless bewilderment and bad attitude. This mother-led episode was the miracle of extended family and cohesive community in the recent but fading past, before cohesive social fabric reverted to paid services performed by strangers. Paid strangers or professional staff are a necessary, even vital, function of the modern world, and yet something has been lost.

Same at home—homemade adaptations as needed, help from family with whatever needed to be dealt with as each day unfolded. Being the fifth of eight kids, Peter had an army of willing help, even before tapping into the extended brood, for which he remains grateful decades later.

The support from family and community made possible the impossible within an educational institution funded to simply make possible the bare minimum of their mandate. Peter and his family had not entertained the high school principal's question *why*; rather, under his mother's leadership they had conspired without compromise to answer, or rather enact, *how*. In 1980, Peter finished high school without missing a beat, graduating with his class—which never happens—and began attending Carleton University the following September. For this next leg of his education, Peter could not bring his friends and extended family to help eliminate barriers as they occurred. Still, Peter embraced the challenge. Good thing; he would be challenged to the core.

Carleton, first a college and later a university, was established in 1942, largely in response to the need to educate returning war veterans, some of whom were disabled, my father among them. In graduating from a college to a university, Carleton needed to expand from its single building in a trendy downtown Ottawa neighbourhood to a large piece of land that would allow for rapid expansion. A large plot of land was purchased in the late 1950s—in those days a move from crowded city to open space being less than two kilometres from the original Carleton College building. The new campus wasn't even going to inconvenience faculty with having to move from their trendy house in the neighbourhood of the old college, called the Glebe.

The new campus included a feature with an unintended consequence. Connecting all buildings on the new campus was an underground tunnel system, designed to shield people from the cold, cruel reality of winter in the Canadian capital. Though unlikely planned with wheelchairs in mind, the tunnel allowed for wheelchair access to all buildings, and being newer buildings, some even had a modicum of accessibility.

Meaning, once inside, the buildings weren't particularly user friendly. New did not make up for poorly conceived building standards, making for difficulties, but not limited to doorways, washrooms, elevators, ramps, or lack thereof. Still, the impossibility of post-secondary education for people with mobility disabilities had shifted to merely highly problematic. Without much else to recommend itself on the accessibility file, by the 1970s Carleton had become the default post-secondary institution of choice for a small but growing student population. And given the state of inaccessibility in transportation, housing, and attendant services then, many of these students decided to live in the poorly accessible residence, over inaccessible everything else, come hell or high water.

When Peter moved into residence in September 1980, the water was high and hell was on its way. Those early pioneering students experienced hardship and privation before staff woke from their complacent slumber and started making changes. It took the tenacity of a core group of students to grind through a degree, and nursing staff in the residence infirmary increasingly were called upon to attend to students without attendants before the university realized that this problem, these students, and the opportunity they presented was not going away. And it *was* an opportunity, though this fact would not become fully understood for several decades. In the absence of accessibility, personal persistence and resourcefulness allowed students to survive, their problem being a bit of an embarrassment to be managed on the periphery of university functioning. Thirty-five years later, and owing to the accomplishments of these accessibility pioneers, the intention to lead in the field of accessibility has become one of Carleton's strategic priorities, enshrined in its strategic plan. It is possibly the first university in the world to have done so.

In the meantime, students struggled. Reflecting back over the decades, Peter matter-of-factly describes a situation he encountered in his first year. And as I write this account I realize that the matter-of-fact, low-key way these young quadriplegics routinely mentioned what amounts to the horrors of their struggle is a constant— constant theme, constant and unconscious show of courage and grace, constant daily fact. Peter is as tough as an old school NHL enforcer and does not have the capacity for self-pity. However difficult or torturous the vicissitudes of life, he simply decides to buck up, shut up, and move on—especially remarkable for those whose constant vicissitude is the inability to move.

With only a limited number of attendants available, briefly morning and nighttime, Peter was sitting for much too long, and his skin broke down. This is a common problem for people with a spinal cord injury, exacerbated by being unable to feel. If not monitored, skin breakdown can progress into an ulcerated gaping wound, become infected, and lead to serious damage or even death. By the time

Peter's skin problem was noticed, it required immediate and decisive action. The problem was, decisive action manifested itself as need for complete inaction. Peter was prescribed to lie on his stomach in bed for two weeks, propped up by pillows, requiring repositioning with the delivery of each meal, these the only three events in an otherwise uneventful day, all day, every day.

Two weeks out of a lifetime doesn't seem so long. Einstein may have conjured his theory of relativity, but Peter came to know the reality of its slow drip. At the time, Peter might have said that it is not relative, that time can stop. The drone of the last second's tick hangs suspended, unable to move events forward, unable to provide relief in the knowledge that at least all things must end.

He had nothing to do. Peter cannot remember why nothing was provided, why he didn't ask. Except for a very few perfunctory minutes each day, Peter was alone. During his brief contact with humanity, he was fed, so talk was limited—one way, if at all. Besides, with nothing happening and the person feeding being one of several disinterested caretakers, real conversation could not happen. Peter had his community back home in Arnprior, only 45 minutes away, and legions would have come had they known, but they did not know. His rock, his mother, would have galvanized a supportive troop into action, but she was away in California. For reasons he is not even sure of, though his unrelenting toughness has to be factored in, he did not let anyone know. Enforcer toughness to a self-injurious fault.

Peter simply decided, without deciding, to endure, as he always has. It is hard to imagine this slow to stoppage of time in the age of distraction: no internet, Netflix, texting, emails, Facebook, e-books, audiobooks, Apple music, human contact— virtual or real—just alone with your thoughts, the same ruminating strains sliding through and rotating back, the narrative wheel becoming more painstaking and disjointed each time it rotates, if it rotates at all. But of course, time does not actually stop; at least that is the theory for those who have not endured Peter's ordeal.

Peter's toughness or stubbornness or drive has served him well throughout his education and in his career. For most of us, it is hard to imagine why we would feel compelled to do something against all odds of success. Life tends to be tough enough without having to prove that we can do the impossible, then get up and do it all over again the next day, and every day for the rest of our lives. Still, this is what he does, and thinks it is nothing to get excited about.

Peter completed his degree at Carleton before renovations made his room accessible, before attendant services made it possible to survive without endless struggle. He then completed a law degree five kilometres down the canal at the University of Ottawa, and he now works full-time as a human rights lawyer in government. He has been asked *why* since returning to high school just after his injury but never sweats the answer to why in pursuit of the answer to *how*, just like his mum.

Peter's habitual matter-of-fact statements about what it took to get an education, forge a career, survive, are never a boast but rather a self-effacing nonchalant admission of strength. The NHL enforcer analogy fits, but the hockey enforcer is playing a role in front of adoring crowds and is being paid big bucks. Peter's strength, toughness, and stoic resilience are the real deal and performed at all times, usually to a crowd of none, without pay—well, at least in this life—more on this point later.

When we talk more than 40 years after his accident, and more than 10 years after his cousin's death, Peter's most heartfelt moment exists in expressing compassion for Terry. Peter and Terry were Ottawa Valley born and bred, both from big Irish Catholic families, and being from a similar brood of nine I can readily identify. We three were lost as middle children, which, combined with our Irish Catholic heritage, is a prescription for the unemotive male, the very epitome of inarticulation. Peter and I fit the stereotype, but Terry, much like Paul Menton, was the exception—a warm guy who wore his heart on his sleeve and, to the extent that disability caused social isolation, was more likely to suffer.

Objectively, Peter's case for sympathy is greater; he has endured more years as a quadriplegic, but that is not how his mind works. I can't imagine the experience of severe disability without the necessity of looking inward severely and often. Peter's immobility cannot constrain his humanity. Which is to say, real strength, even beyond the ability to absorb pain, is the ability to transcend the cards we are dealt. Few of us do it substantially; those few do it unceasingly.

Foreknowledge of what quadriplegia meant coupled with his habit of falling asleep at the wheel that had caused his accident did not make Terry's adjustment easier. Waking into the nightmare of his sun-filled hospital room, Terry was suspended between disbelief and shame. Nice, sensitive, happy-go-lucky Terry knew too much, and although Peter and Terry remained close, they were never as close as they had been before Terry's accident.

At some level, Terry, and perhaps most injured risk takers, feels he deserves what he got, even as he inwardly screams, *Why me?* One of the nurses on the spinal cord unit once casually said to me that she thought that *they got* what they deserved. She thought that sympathy was misplaced for young guys whose lives were ruined by 30 seconds of inattention or by momentary lapses of judgment. The reason why she worked on a spinal cord unit remained a deep, unfathomable mystery, but not one worth solving. No one should be judged by a spontaneous action at the age of 19. Many of us make bad judgments our whole lives without serious consequences (even atheism is forgivable). In addition to the physical burden of quadriplegia, young people should not have to wear the mark of Cain. That nurse was wrong; her nonchalant cruel assessment, unforgivable.

What actually happens to these young people, mostly guys, is beyond physical loss. The metamorphosis from testosterone-driven, the world is your oyster, all things physical, to complete immobility, future unfathomable, familiar world no longer a place in which you reside, cannot be accounted for or summed up with trite phrases or pop psychology. None of these guys would have chosen, could have brought themselves to understand, what of necessity they were going to have to do, to have to become, just to cope. Those denied a life—that is, from an outside perspective—worth living most often found a life nonetheless. In pulling a life from the ashes, in surviving this minute to the next, 60 times in an hour, 24 hours in a day, endurance can reveal a higher self. This is not necessarily the language of the people I have had the privilege of knowing, but it is what I have witnessed. I know that it happens; I just don't know how.

In 1989, Tom Cruise starred in *Born on the Fourth of July*, based on the novel by Ron Kovic. It is the story of a young guy injured in the Vietnam War and of his difficulty reintegrating back into life as a quadriplegic. It is not an awarding-winning performance, but there is one scene—poignant and raw—when the character breaks down and cries, "But who will love me?" It is *the* question, the one that remains after knowing who will feel sympathy, who will admire, who will support. Answers to the other questions are important and can form the basis of human connection, but they do not answer the inarticulate speech of the heart, which is ultimately a yearning for love.

On the rehab unit we witnessed many couples struggling with their relationship in dealing with a broken spine and broken hearts. When one member of the couple becomes disabled, "through sickness and in health" sadly does not always hold. Promises made, quite apart from the words said, also lie broken.

The chances are better for couples who meet post injury. Expectations are more closely aligned, and the couple is aware of and accepts what they are getting into, with the possibility of deep love following in the wake of seeing each other as they actually are. Still, for all relationships there is uncertainty, and those limitations once accepted must be contended with for the duration.

Vulnerability can also make us look for love in all the wrong places. After Terry's girlfriend left him to go to school, he was alone for some time. Then he fell in love with a nursing student, so who better to know what she was getting into? She accepted his limitations just as she benefited from Terry's warm and loving nature. Still, Terry wanted to sweeten the bargain for the cash-strapped student, his one true love, the one who had finally come into his life to make him whole again. She moved into Terry's apartment and stayed for the duration of her education, which Terry paid for. Then, with education complete, she left, debt-free and free of Terry. She left to pursue her own life, the one that had just opened up, the world, her oyster, hers for the taking. Terry's life, the one that had continued to hold out for the possibility of love in a life that seemed to be defined by loss, closed up, just as he always knew it would, if only he hadn't been sucked into thinking there was hope where none existed.

Terry loved but was unloved; well, it would be more accurate to say Terry was much loved but not by the girl he loved. Peter was never fooled by the girl who broke Terry's heart, and he still bristles at the thought. But Peter's soft spot, his ability to feel deep compassion for his cousin—even if he doesn't seem to feel much of the same for himself—betrays a depth of feeling far beyond the notion of toughness. Peter speaks of deep admiration for his cousin, who let people in, who dared to love, who opened his heart in a way Peter did not, could not, do.

For all Terry's pain and vulnerability for allowing love in and his own comparative safety by refusing to do the same, Peter credits his cousin for a life well-lived. Peter did what he did to be successful in life and is not a creature of regret but understands that articulation of the heart includes the expression of love. And it occurs to me that crediting, admiring, his cousin for the strength to love, regardless of outcome, is actually an admission of love, arrived at in the only way—circuitous, indirect—we unemotive Irish males can manage. I left Peter's apartment that oppressive winter afternoon wishing that he would give himself a break.

Earlier, in a meandering discussion about his life, we had come to the inevitable question about the existence of God. Peter is agnostic, suspended, could go either way, but then quite suddenly he makes a stark declaration: "Even if God does exist, he isn't interested in me." Until that moment, I had been arguing in favour of God on the basis of science, logic, the existence of consciousness, my rational self in full flight. But to this experiential declaration, I had no answer.

God is not a theory, an abstraction, an idea whose time has come or has passed. If God is, God is everywhere, is everything, is one and indivisible. Still, I could not answer, let alone satisfy Peter, nor myself, that God has been, is, will be, interested in him, or any of us. I could not say, let alone believe, at least in that moment, that there is a personal God who is in communion in any personal way with Peter.

Where was Peter's personal God when he was alone in his room in residence for those two weeks of eternity? It wasn't *just* about Peter, but about Peter the question of pain, loss, and suffering loomed large, could not be made trite, could not be explained away. Peter does not do trite, does not make statements to evoke sympathy, is incapable of histrionics. His 45 years of slogging through each day would make it tough for a saint to conclude that God was interested in him, and it was remarkable that Peter did not say the words that hung suspended between us—*he could not believe, because he had been abandoned by God.*

And for this reason, that is, my inability to arrive at an answer that I would not be embarrassed by, could have faith in, I stopped writing this book for two years. Well, I didn't so much decide to stop as, unable to answer Peter, I was unable to continue. I often returned to the question of a personal God but could not quite formulate an answer that did not have a whiff of condescension. However I might respond, I could not speak to Peter's experience, and much as I do not like the term *appropriating voice*, I had to admit that almost anything I might say would do just that. Peter's heartfelt, stoically delivered bottom line about his life, and a thousand others I've had the privilege of knowing, leaves me flat and despondent. Who can argue with Peter's low-key unemotional conclusion that he was abandoned by God? Who, after all, deals the cards we are required to live with? Hard to argue for a dispassionate God, the dealer; harder still a personal God who knows you, is interested in you, loves you, and—the most powerful indictment—feels compassion for you. What does Peter say in prayer to a personal God who did this to him, personally?

It remains depressingly true that the notion of a personal God as relates to the reality of pain, loss, and death may be the most compelling reason *not* to believe. Still, and stated with the luxury of not having had to face what Peter has had to face, difficult challenge in itself does not prove or disprove the existence of God; it proves rather our all too human bewilderment at what and where God's intention leads to. The driving force of this book, mostly ruminated on during my 3 a.m. angst-ridden pondering, is that the passive nihilistic pablum that is being swallowed as never before as a distinguishing feature of modernity is not good enough.

Time passes. Sitting, thinking, one summer afternoon at a cottage near Algonquin Park, I happened to reread a piece Peter had written some years earlier about the first moments of his accident. And as often happens in life, I realized that my first view had been blind; that is, I had taken in the words but had not seen, absorbed, what they meant. Peter essentially answered my question in his recollection, and in doing so exposed a level of insight and sensitivity that is not so much surprising as it is profound.

> The blow was of such force I was stunned, but only momentarily. I understood immediately the peril I faced. I knew I had to roll over or die. But I was powerless. I could not move. The circuitry was blown. So I held my breath. It was all I could do. Time passed, seemingly years, decades, centuries. I had reached the apex ... my lungs were bursting. I knew I was about to die. There was no panic. Rather, a transcendent calm came over me. *I've had a good life,* I thought, *but now it's over.* And in that millisecond I accepted death, I became hyper aware of everything that had ever transpired in my life. It did not pass before my eyes temporally in the manner of a high speed film. On the contrary, the temporal no longer mattered. Time had ceased to exist. In the barest interlude between life and death, omniscience was the rule. My birth, my joys, my disappointments, my loves, my heartaches ... all were experienced contemporaneously with a previously unmatched intensity. I was at peace, totally content. The constraints of time were broken. I had achieved infinity. And then I rolled over. To once again feel the gentle caress of the June sun on my face was the most powerful moment of my young life. Oh, I grasped the seriousness of my fall. I knew without thinking its probable outcome. But to come face to face with death, indeed, to truly comprehend the utter finality of death is to garner an unparalleled love of life. Thinking I was messin' around, my friend Jim had playfully turned me over from my dead man's float and looked down upon me laughing at what seemed to be a

hilariously classic wipeout. Little did he know he had pulled me back from the abyss. Even so, in that profoundly joyous moment, I still could not breathe. My lungs were full of water. I could sense the fear lapping at the edge of my consciousness. I frantically struggled to lift my arms, move my legs to breathe. Something. Anything. I fought to break through the numbness. Nothing. "Don't panic, Pete," my dad's voice warmly flooded over me, "don't panic." He was with me though miles away. My dad's pride calmed me. *I won't die, Dad*, I thought, *I'm too strong*.

Focusing on Jim's eyes, I looked at him ... reaching, willing him to understand something had gone very, very wrong. "Get Mike," I spat, water and sand screwing from my mouth, "get Mike!" Suddenly comprehending the danger, Jim's face took on a look of confusion and horror that will remain with me always. "Mike," he screamed, "Mike!" All hell broke loose. In the bedlam, people were jumping into the water surrounding me shouting and crying. I could see their hands reaching for me though I felt nothing. I coughed and sputtered ... more water, more sand spewing forth. Looking up into the faces of friends I had known my entire life, however, I felt momentarily safe. "Get Mum," I repeated over and over, "she's at the beach." My friends were with me. They would take care of me. I would be O.K. Maybe I could relax, but just for a minute. Almost seductively, something stronger than the paralyzingly numbness overtaking my body was consuming my will. In the cacophony of shouting and screaming an unnatural fatigue was pulling me from the familiar faces above. They grew distant. My sight was fading. The sun crowded everything from my vision. Confusion seeped in. I no longer recognized my rescuers. My eyelids fluttered and I thought, *I'll just close my eyes*. I needed to close my eyes. So I did. My ears were ringing incessantly. Flat, toneless but increasing in power. My senses were overwhelmed yet the soothing scent of Mum's perfume lingered. "Stay with me Peter, stay with me," I heard a voice commanding me ... a lifeguard's voice ... so professional, so calm. "Don't go, Pete," implored another. "Pete," another voice cried, reaching into my very core. "Peter," I heard her pleading. "It's Mum. Wake up, Pete. Hold on." My eyes snapped open. An upside-down face was looking into mine. Confused, I didn't understand. And then, in an instant, clarity reasserted my harsh reality. "Stay with me, Peter," Mike kept repeating, his arms on both sides of my head stabilizing my neck. I could see Mum's face. Distraught, she looked so beaten. Her spirit crushed. "I broke my neck," the words spilled out as I chastised myself for being weak and bringing my Mum such grief. She was crying. I could not bear it. An ethereal quiet descended upon us. We were alone. Looking into eyes, smiling, I whispered, "I'm alright, Mum," with a false bravado disconnected from the terror percolating just below the surface. But I wasn't, and the anguished look on my Mum's face told me she was well aware. It haunts me still.

Peter's recollection decades after the accident is far more than just an impressive recall of detail. Peter's narrative is *infused* with a personal God, even as he suggests that he was abandoned. This juxtaposition is neither contradiction nor semantics; Peter's experience is his own—and yet, we, all of us, are not only free to extract meaning from whomever God places in our path; we are required to do so, even if the passivity of modern life has seduced us into thinking otherwise.

At the beginning of his summer holidays, a rambunctious boy at the tender age of 15 has a terrible accident and immediately thinks, *I've had a good life, and now it's over*. Why? Because "a transcendent calm came over me." Peter writes that before being pulled back to the physical realm by his dad's warm voice and his mum's "pleading," "I was at peace, totally content. The constraints of time were broken. I had achieved infinity." Such are the words of a spiritual sage, rather than an action-oriented testosterone-driven teenager, and I don't doubt for a second that Peter experienced these insights and emotions. What I do doubt is the modern view of Peter's transcendent experience as simply a neurological event.

And what is the modern view of transcendent experience? We moderns have replaced doubt and wonder with cynical certainty even as the certainty of our cynicism is simply capitulation to death. Weirdly, human fear can lead us to embrace the very thing that we fear most, an ennui-driven version of Stockholm syndrome—that is, acceptance of oblivion as escape from ambiguity.

The question may not be Why do we die? but rather Why do we live? I have always had a hard time feeling the presence of God in and of my own thoughts and experiences, but it is precisely because of the spectacular lives of others—including spectacularly painful and Peter-esque tough aspects to life—that I have something to cling on to, something that cannot be explained or explained away, something that resembles faith. My two years of inertia were born of the fact that I have not lived Peter's life, and his experience once lived might change my perspective. Still, I can only go with what I've got, and I am not judging his experience, rather am inspired by it, even if he is unimpressed. To my warped version of our short sojourn, lives have meaning, some more than others, and perhaps Peter's most of all, however contrary to anyone's choosing his experience might be. I know this is a controversial thought, and I am not suggesting that we value one person's life more than any other, but it does seem obvious that some people, whether or not of their choosing, imprint humanity writ large, exposing courage, great integrity, and sacrifice, consequently inspiring love, gratitude, and compassion. Most people, in aspiring to comfort and safety, seem determined to leave no tracks or imprint at all. So, to Peter's bottom line statement/question, my pathetic bottom line answer is that he rips open the facade of life frivolously lived by most, exposing meaning for those who care to see.

Discussion about the existence of God makes people uncomfortable. It has become a social norm, for which there is heavy expectation, to properly genuflect to modernity by stating allegiance to the nothingness of atheism. Still, in looking at empirical science, I like God's chances. Looking at the logic of intention and design we have a strong case, thank you, Mr. Flew. But there is more. More personal, more subjective, and more compelling. Consciousness is our vessel for inferring meaning, and its ability to interpret, synthesize, and know is far greater than the analysis of logical data. Dawkins's work ignores the deep-seated intelligence of our archetypal selves—that shared source of the profound, that non-scientific place from which we experience love, grief, beauty, and yes, if we are connected to our higher selves, awe. Khalil Gibran captures the concept in a few words: "When you reach the end of what you should know, you will be at the beginning of what you should sense."

Comfort will not reveal meaning. The extremity of human existence—Peter's accident, Terry's abandonment, the lives and deaths of my all-too-human cast of characters—is where the essence and meaning of life, beyond the physical exterior, may be momentarily glimpsed. I can't say why or how exactly, but what we come to suspect or even know does not always come neatly packaged with empirical bows. Still, I maintain that my magnificent characters are far more than the pain and isolation of temporal experience, and their daily grind exists as an example of accessing a higher self in a life well—or even spectacularly—lived.

Thus, if we consciously open our eyes and use consciousness in place of distraction, if we take personally the experience of whomever is placed on our path, we might begin to see the semblance of a personal God. Most of us, most of the time, hang suspended, uncertain, and, significantly, unwilling to decide. The societal forces of negation and disbelief are much more pervasive today than having and holding faith. Belief takes real strength, and where doubt exists it is much easier to take the path of least resistance, even if it doesn't lead anywhere. Both literally and metaphorically, the road that leads over the cliff and to our waiting demise is the default road most travelled. And even as we anticipate our free-floating lemming-like fate, we mostly do so without question. Life as such is not a metamorphosis but rather a societal pact trading fear for collective amnesia. Avoidance will not deliver us from what must come.

At some level we know that the beauty, complexity, pain, and longing of our experience cannot be reduced to biological cellular functioning. We know, but we keep the passive acceptance of Dawkins's brave new world separate from the stuff of dreams of our waking consciousness. The people I write about are not variations on an amoeba; our ability to soar through time and space, seeking communion in the consciousness of others, is not a trifle. Consciousness is the conduit from humanity to divinity, from impersonal to personal. It is not about whether or not we have mobility; it is not about the body at all. For all the reasons not to believe, there is the miracle of consciousness—that non-physical, ultra-mobile, spiritual entity we experience out of body at will, and for all the modernist attempts to explain it away, it cannot be explained or accounted for by any material measure, and never will be. We know this; we just don't have faith in what we know.

I think, therefore I am not simply biology.

I think, therefore Richard Dawkins is not right.

I think, therefore I am not nothing that came from nothing that will come to nothing.

I think,

You think,

I am,

We are.

Chapter Eight

"I DON'T WANT TO MISS A THING"

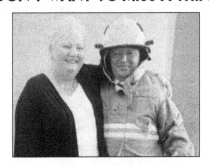

*"I don't want to fall asleep
'Cause I'd miss you, babe
And I don't want to miss a thing."*
Aerosmith (1998)

It was her favourite song, I was to learn, later. It was a popular song by Aerosmith, I was to learn, later. Funny, the things you don't know about people that you know. We worked together for 15 years. She was my work wife, my wife kidded—that is, with me for 40 daytime hours each week, compared, to say, a half that for the wife I was married to. I knew her best and not at all. Janice elevated work from mundane to spectacular just by being her plain old self.

A vice-president I worked for and kidded with once asked, "Why is university politics so fierce?" to which he answered with a mildly facetious truism: "Because nothing that matters ever happens here."

Still, my version is that the work we did to get students with disabilities basic accommodations mattered a lot. Years ago, the faculty response to providing accommodations required by legislation was uneven, or arbitrary, requiring us to use our most advanced Fuller Brush salesperson techniques. There were many skirmishes along the way, and getting faculty to take us seriously was always an effort. Still, the decades churned, resistance lessened, faculty mostly came around, and accommodating students with disabilities became a regular part of how the university conducted its business.

Although providing accommodations such as extra time or a quiet location to write exams was the controversial part, the often-ignored pieces that helped students most were the skill development and guidance from their coordinator. This student development aspect, anchored in the therapeutic alliance, is why our students with disabilities went from significant probability of failure to beating the general population 7-year graduation rate over a 20-year period. It is a big deal in the post-secondary sector to move the graduation rate up a percentage or two for the general population. A 20 percent increase in 20 years for our cohort of students with significant obstacles is considered impossible. And yet that is what they did.

Future outcomes will be interesting. Today a wide swath of students with poor mental health is registering with our centre. Some have diagnosed psychiatric disabilities, and some are fragile young people who suffer from a generalized inability to cope with the demands of life. In recent years, human rights thinking has stripped away disability offices' ability to effectively differentiate between demonstrable disability-related need, based on assessment and diagnosis, and any number of academic or emotional difficulties. If articulating this concern seems like tough talk, the opposite is closer to the truth.

Our intent and actions are dedicated to the students' best interest by getting to the heart of the matter rather than assuming everyone has similar needs. Some students need accommodations, and no amount of remedial help will change that, while others need skill development and/or regular contact with someone who knows them, cares about them, and can act as their anchor in the tidal currents of university demands. If we don't do the hard work, if we simply give everyone what they believe they need based on rights thinking, students can be burdened by choice, are more likely to flounder, less likely to graduate.

While human rights thinking may apply to the post-secondary sector, an uncompromising rights mindset causes problems once individuals leave college and university in search of a career. Jobs are won by those who metaphorically kick down the door and declare their ability to contribute, and not by those whose interview strategy is to first inform the perspective employer of their needs. Someone who can convince an employer of their drive to contribute in their first volley can easily work in their needs on the tail end of a successful pitch.

All of which is to say that the reception area outside our cozy closed office doors became increasingly rancorous over the years. For all the work that happens with professional coordinators behind closed doors, the real drama and often best work happens in the mosh pit of reception. That was Janice's domain, and in this jungle of anxious bodies, cramped space, and competing interests, her rule was absolute. Parenthetically, when asked over the years why our slice of humanity seemed to run so well, despite the impossibility of its task, my answer has always been "I have one skill: hiring the right people." Never more so than with Janice.

Janice's most distinguishing feature was her laugh. It was an eruption of piercing noise, irreverence, and spontaneous joy. It was exactly as she was, and it is why I hired her. Not only that, I recruited her, though I didn't know her. I only knew that laugh and its effect on people. She had been across campus working in health and counselling services, another unforgiving heaven or hell hole of human activity—hell to most, heaven to Janice. Much of life is how we choose to interpret the cards we are dealt, and I wanted the Janice effect rubbing off on our crew. Poaching staff is not exactly encouraged, but I didn't care. I had a job opening, so I called her and said, "You don't know me but ..." and proceeded to make an offer she could have refused but, to my everlasting gratitude, did not. And so, history began.

It was a good move for her. Less formal, more room for discretion, or in her case indiscretion, more weirdos—and that's just the staff, whom she always endearingly referred to as her "peeps."

It was a great move for us, adding someone with combustible transformative powers, capable of massaging fear or anger or crisis into humour or shared moment or hope. And really, what could be healthier than detaching ourselves from the narrow suffocating of the subjectivity of our life as tragedy for the shared continuous belly laugh of life that was Janice's life. Easy concept, but tough to pull off, toughest yet to inspire in others. But she did it, every day for 15 years.

Absolutely everyone knew Janice, which did not make her a social butterfly. On the contrary she seemed to have an authentic relationship with all her peeps and vastly extended family. Wherever I went people would ask me to pass on my regards to Janice, which, as Louis Armstrong croons in "What a Wonderful World," is just another way of saying "I love you."

And despite being out of tune with university expectations of discretion, sensitivity, and virtue-signalling conformity—which Janice didn't do—she didn't have an enemy in the world. Not conforming to the fiction of tolerance in a sector becoming increasingly intolerant is dangerous, but she didn't notice or didn't care. Our office dealt in serious problems mostly—all the more reason to apply the antidote to life's challenges: irreverent humour at full volume without a care in the world, even as her audience giggled and glanced about the room for fear of offended parties.

The only explanation for how she got away with it was that laugh. Every hour of every day from some quarter of our centre over all the noise from other quarters came that familiar true surround-sound, the DNA of PMC, floating over and above, a virtuosity, the Stradivarius of laughing instruments, the glue and structure of every day, the most constant feature of our working life.

There was also that morale thing. Work was fun, funny, and productive, engaged with the people you liked best, no separation between work and leisure, just more meaning—meaning that you could never retire, because it could never, ever end. Even, or especially, the mundane or inconvenient details of work became an opportunity to work her irreverent magic. One among many examples was the temporary occupation that almost became a permanent resettlement. Our fluid space situation required that Janice temporarily move in with and share an office with Bruce, both of them now across the hall from my office. The full pageantry of what followed was mine to take in for eight or more hours each day.

Bruce is a quiet guy, and his office time had been quiet until the temporary occupation. Janice considered it her right to never be quiet and was determined that Bruce would agree with her. Bruce agreed with her to keep her quiet, but that didn't work. Janice decided that since she and Bruce shared a space they should logically share their marital bonds—that is, Janice made Bruce her work husband, delighted us with her bawdy interpretation of what that means, and proceeded to make Bruce's life miserable. No human being had conjured sexual innuendo out of every spoken word until Janice married Bruce without a ceremony but with that laugh and orders to "shut your gob" whenever he meekly attempted to temper the honeymoon for that pesky thing called work. Good thing Bruce was a good sport.

Oddly, Janice's impression of herself was somewhat different than how Bruce and I and, well, everyone else saw her. She saw herself as shy and retiring (while always adding that she never intended to actually retire) and not a shrieking madwoman capable of talking faster than an auctioneer. Which is why one Monday morning I challenged her, and she took the bait. I made a wager to Janice in front of her peeps that she could not remain silent for the entirety of one full work week. Easy-peasy, she responded, and then she proceeded to cram as many words into the conversation as she could before the official moratorium on making noise began.

Of course, we all knew I would win, and everyone, especially Bruce, luxuriated in the silence that was beyond golden during that brief time while Janice's painful resolve held (which didn't prevent her from spending a good part of the day sitting on Bruce's lap). Though we couldn't admit it, we were surprised and impressed that hours ticked by without laughter, with steely silence pervading the corridors and offices of our centre. It was eerily other people's normal, a state of being we had never actually experienced.

Still, the quiet air was electric with happening. All morning she held fast, with only her handwritten notes asking us to "shut our gobs" as evidence of her desire to communicate. We whispered and giggled like grade-schoolers watching Janice struggle against silence and would not have been surprised if smoke came out of her ears. We could not quite believe that for all her struggle—bearing in mind that Janice was what you would call single-minded—she was doing exactly what *we* wanted. We—primarily Bruce—savoured that one day like a fine wine, while Janice considered making a case for torture to the United Nations, or so she said when our golden delight unceremoniously came to an end. At noon that first day she erupted with laughter, with outrage, with full volume heart and soul Janice, and it was over.

Funny thing is, once the need of temporary office occupation ended, neither Janice nor Bruce wanted their own office. Which puzzled me, so I asked Janice. At which point she dramatically jumped on, or back onto, Bruce's lap and claimed she could not live a second without him. Bruce merely shrugged his shoulders as if resigned, but I knew he loved every second, and while she had been silent, he had actually missed that laugh. Janice's bluster and noisy chaos was actually artistry of the highest order, pulling people from themselves into what they wanted to be. And most people really do want to be the type of person who has fun. Serious as this world may be, we do want to have fun, and we gravitate to those who include us, shy and retiring as we may be, into the party that never ends.

Of course, the party is just cover for the depth of human emotion rattling below the surface of all human interaction; it is a trick, permission, the key to the lock of our inarticulation that we want to reveal, that we want known.

But we don't talk of such things; we just kind of rejoice without question in the midst of the one who unlocks. And for she who unlocks and never shuts up, questions are never tolerated, party poopers not allowed. Weirdly, in this caldron of articulating gobs and faux marital bliss, both Janice and Bruce actually got a lot of work done. Seriously. Turns out I was a productivity guru and didn't know it. The management secret was to harness that force of nature, which was a force both natural and beyond nature, called Janice.

Parties help with the illusion of forever but cannot go on forever. Our Hurricane Janice, Tasmanian devil of constant swirling energy, the literal and figurative life of the party, was human after all. She got sick. Bladder cancer. Some treatment but not chemo, yet. She was the epitome of optimism—didn't know any other way to be—and everyone knows that being positive in life is how you defeat cancer.

Cancer spreads. From bladder to kidney. More optimism. You only need one kidney, after all.

Aggressive treatment; same result. Surgically reconstructed bladder and removal of kidney, with chemo to follow. That should do it. As soon as possible she wanted to visit us, being unhappy to be away from work, determined to be back at work as soon as possible, which she intended to be faster than was humanly possible. Her doctors did not share her optimism. They wanted Janice to change her status from sick leave to long-term disability—that is, reconcile herself to the fact that it ain't happening.

While the work situation hangs suspended, we prepare for her visit, unsure what to expect. It's been some months, and we all know cancer changes people. We guiltily suspect that maybe we overdid the fun, life being serious and sad after all. We organize a breakfast, 8 a.m., a table full of anxious people, Janice understandably a few minutes late. She approaches from the long corridor, and our table goes silent, watching. Janice walks to our table full stride, plants her feet, wide smile as she shouts "Ta da" and dramatically pulls off a purple wig to reveal her baby bottom-esque scalp, pink, bare, and more naked than seems possible. And she laughs, that familiar sound of home, chortling with effect, not a smidgen of self-consciousness in surely one of the heaviest, most poignant moments in life—that is, for the rest of us. Our gal is back.

Janice always did take life by the humorous horns. Still, even when she did do something to be the centre of attention, which was always, it was not actually about her. She desperately wanted *everyone* to share in the joke, no exceptions, in the holy, humorous moment, most often at the expense of self and not about self. Her outrageous, habitual, attention-seeking behaviour was literally unselfish. I forgot to tell her that.

Doctors be damned, she comes back to work. It's been a year, and we are thrilled. Her courage alone attests to the strength of human will, and we harbour the illusion that the centre will hold. But you learn in life that the centre cannot hold easily, naturally, or permanently. We are all on borrowed time, borrowed place, borrowed happiness. Who or what we think we are is not for long. It isn't just gratitude we lack—though we are sorely lacking in that—it is awareness of just how bloody spectacularly exceptional the existence of life is within a universe too vast and hostile to life to comprehend. Janice lived life as exceptional, and we were witnesses, and she fooled us into believing that it was commonplace and sustainable. We don't contemplate life, the universe, our own small existence, or the singularity of Janice often enough.

We all participate in life's conspiracy. We dwell within a necessary fiction about where it all leads—maybe a certain amount of denial is needed so that we don't take ourselves too seriously. Plausible deniability keeps us from being too morbid to live, I suppose—but the trick is to not to swallow the death-denying cult of modernity. Living life well with knowledge of the certainty of death is either a fine line of possibility or else the ultimate oxymoron, which Janice just happened to finesse with the poetic touch of Shakespeare, or even Aerosmith.

For more than two years Janice did everything right, submitting to dehumanizing treatments, enduring sickness, pain, baldness, and exposure. She maintained hope, though none was forthcoming from her doctors, which, objectively speaking, must be a very large red flag. We had loved having her back at work, but it didn't last long. She developed a low-grade persistent cough, no big deal until the diagnosis of lung cancer. Even this, of the poor prognosis cancer category, she endured with a smile, intent on beating every and all of life's vicissitudes with proper treatment and improper resolve. She didn't know what else to do. She was not one for defeat. There had to be a joke in this.

Months passed. A group of us, say six or eight, sat at Somei's (another of Janice's long-time peeps) house after dinner and much ribald humour. Particularly ribald because Paddy Stewart (close friend and comedic entertainer at seniors' homes) had brought his kilted boy doll Fergus, whose most distinguishing feature was his autonomically inappropriately incorrect pink-hued Celtic penis. Janis insisted on both holding and holding onto Fergus as we sat, and, strange as it might seem, it was the perfect moment. Forget the pink penis; it was perfect as in the right people in harmony at a precise moment locked in time forever. I'm not being clever—I actually believe that memory, longing, these moments, may be a portal to time in perpetuity, perfection, a hint of what is vaguely referred to as heaven.

We, of course, perfected perfection by retelling Gord Paynter's punchline, lifting Fergus's kilt and declaring in our best Scottish brogue, "Put your hand up again and see if it grew some more!" Each time the punchline is reiterated, we all laugh as if heard for the first time. Okay, so perfect moment for idiots, but we still claim it as such because we are with those we love, and since we laugh so as not to cry, we laugh again and again. Our laugh articulates our sense of futility and sadness about the fact that Janice is dying. Crying is not allowed, and there is nothing we can do.

That is, until Janice speaks up. "You know," she begins, uncharacteristically casual, almost circumspect, "Eddie [lifetime live-in squeeze of 23 years] and I never did get married, which is too bad." Brief and rare silence, thoughts dripping with possibility and intent, the echo of Janice's words percolating into resolve. Our mission was born. We were not going to be funeral dwellers; we were going to be wedding planners!

If ever there was an example that opposites attract, it would be the relationship between exuberant Janice and her much maligned, eternally willing to be the butt of all jokes, partner, Eddie. Being a good sport was an essential quality for being in a relationship with Janice. Best example: Janice loved, er, lusted after hunky firemen in their firefighting work clothes. She loved their trucks, their hoses, the fact that they slide down a pole; there were many, many ways Janice publicly declared her fetish for firemen, and Eddie bore a thousand cutting comparisons to uniformed firemen with saintly forbearance. And we loved Eddie too, and not just his willingness to suffer. We knew money was the reason they hadn't married, but we were determined that it was not going to be the reason they didn't marry now. And, left unsaid, Janice didn't have much time.

Next day, we roared into action, and by week's end our plan was substantially in place. We started with a little white lie, telling Janice that the wedding had to happen in April instead of her preferred June, because of the availability of facilities. She had wanted warm weather and fresh flowers in bloom; we wanted her alive and feeling well enough to enjoy the moment. In consideration of money and in order to be able to gather all her peeps, we conspired to hold the wedding at the university. Funny thing happened. Janice's name opened doors, opened wallets, opened hearts. Turns out there are advantages to not having enemies. Most important, we were able to book the grand hall: big open space, high ceilings, and beautiful views of the river. After that, refreshments, sound equipment, chairs, set-up, flowers—all donated, including people volunteering for the event, their excuse being that they wouldn't miss it for the world.

Then there was music. The great hall has a valuable donated grand piano that is under the auspices of the chair of the music department. He, Dr. James Wright, is a world-class pianist and composer whom I just happened to know. And he of course knew Janice, thereby nullifying his need to know me. Many obligations, difficult timing due to him being on sabbatical and away, but merely a moment's hesitation before his absolute commitment.

Now what is a world-class piano played by a world-class pianist lacking? A world-class soprano, of course. The previous summer I'd met a young woman busking in the downtown market. She was remarkable because she sang complex, challenging arias, while seemingly impervious to the background of bustling people, barking dogs, and traffic. I have to admit she had me with her first few piercing notes from my favourite aria, "O Mio Babbino Caro." She was beauty and bustle in the midst of discordant market sounds, which I just happened to record. Which turned out well, because once I played James a clip, he said he wanted to meet and work with her. Though that hadn't happened, I still had her card, and I called to see if she was interested in a busking performance in front of several hundred people. Marie Claire had moved from Ottawa but immediately agreed to come back and perform for Janice's wedding. She had never met Janice, but, like everyone else, she was prey to the irresistible compulsion that was pulling this unlikely event together.

Attendance at an event does not give much away regarding how bloody complicated they can be to organize. Linda, Amanda, and Jocelyn stepped up and took over the heavy lifting. They had organized a few successful events for our office but were not wedding planners—weddings having a special set of challenges, sensitivities, and ways to get into trouble. They instantly became wedding planners extraordinaire. To this day I marvel at why people plan weddings a year in advance. Seems about 51 weeks too long.

Needless to say, with about six weeks planning, we were ahead of schedule, and not for lack of complexity. This was going to be Janice's wedding, the one she never had, and knowing she was dying was going to make it poignant, meaningful, and potentially sombre as hell. None of us wanted to deny this reality, but we needed something else in our wedding planning arsenal—something particular to Janice and yet something that would include the forgotten groom. After all, the phenomenon of Janice cast a big shadow. Eddie was content to take a back seat in this, and in all things, but given the size of Janice's personality, I was afraid he might end up in the trunk.

Then I had a thought. People who know me always say this is a dangerous moment; some say a moment they hope never comes. I called a friend and former colleague who had left us and moved on to Toronto for, of all things, a man. At her engagement party the previous year I had met her uncle, who was an area fire chief. He gave me the number of a volunteer group of firemen who came to worthy public events. My request was a bit unusual, the volunteer coordinator acknowledged; in fact it had never been asked for before. Undeterred, I continued.

It was great that four firemen volunteered to come to the wedding in a fire truck and in their formal uniforms. Still, we all knew Janice's fetish was specifically tethered to the firefighting garb and not the formal uniform. I considered explaining this nuanced reality to my volunteer coordinator but thought he might get the wrong idea. With trepidation I asked, in addition to the four formal firemen and official firetruck, would there be any chance that they could possibly bring old grimy fire duds and boots for one short, aging, slightly plumpish groom?

The volunteer coordinator was an agreeable guy, so his perplexity was understated, but clearly, he didn't get it. I continued that Janice had an attraction to firemen, an attraction that the groom had put up with for 23 years, and so for just this one day, their wedding day, could we arrange for Eddie, disparaged by Janice's many ogling jokes, to be transformed into the object of her desire? Without necessarily getting what I was talking about still, the agreeable volunteer said, oh sure, and it was done.

The day before the wedding, Janice had the audacity to ask if she had any input into music. *How ungrateful!* we thought. Truth is, she and Eddie were mostly happy for us to make the arrangements—they had other, more important, matters to attend to. Most of all, their job was to make sure Janice was rested up enough to be able to enjoy herself at her wedding, the one that was only going to happen because of the illness that caused her to need to rest up. Janice wanted us to play a recording of Aerosmith's "Don't Want to Miss a Thing" as she walked down the aisle. I can't claim to be an Aerosmith fan, though I'd definitely include myself in the not-an-Aerosmith-fan category. Still, I had to conclude even before hearing their whiney classic that the title was Janice-perfect.

All of which was making for an interesting program. In the days leading up to the wedding there was a collective buzz. It wasn't just that people, campus departments, and neighbourhood stores donated, well, everything. Alta Vista Flowers called, insisting to be part of the action. The owner had never met Janice but had experienced her laugh over the phone. A professional photographer no one knew heard about the coming nuptials and asked if he could be the wedding photographer for free. Expressionless people I had passed in the corridors for years suddenly became animated and personable and begged to be allowed to attend. That would be the wee wedding a few friends decided to put on for a friend that morphed into the social event of the century.

In addition to those who begged to attend were the invited guests, many of whom had scheduling conflicts since we only got around to making a guest list two weeks before the wedding. Still, we ended up with a 100 percent attendance rate. People knew you just had to be there. Why? Most human events, including or perhaps especially weddings, evoke mixed feelings towards the recipients of attention. Our human event had no ambiguity. Everyone was pulling in the same direction in a way that rarely happens today. Common values, that thing that used to rally people into unity and togetherness, is all but absent in a modern individual-rights world that disparages the notion of common as too common and well past. It isn't, and these rare glimpse into human potential by way of human tragedy prove that people still want to articulate as one voice from the same bleeding-heart hymnbook.

Back to the program, moments before it was about to begin. The great hall was perfect—having people in life really does help. I have no idea how most of the decorations and arrangements were made; I just know that Jocelyn and Amanda worked their magic. The antique grand piano had been wheeled out of storage and positioned in full view beside the living plant wall and the most spectacle wood sculpture in the world. To which there is a history. About 25 years ago, I sought out the guy whose sculptures adorned our campus. I had to know who had created these impossibly curvaceous complex pieces that took the breath away from the odd person like me, while remaining unnoticed by many. David Fels and I met and, having in common our love of wood, quickly became friends.

A few years back, I was walking in a park near my house with my two trusty Portuguese water dogs. I noticed that our much loved 200-year-old oak residing near the Rideau River was dying. Next day I asked two questions; to David I asked, Would you want to carve this unique tree? And to the city, Do you have plans for this tree once it is cut down? David said yes in an instant, and the city said no, though the question had to be asked for some months before we received an answer. David Barkley, head arborist (no joke), then took an interest and had the tree carcass delivered to the university, where it was transformed into the magnificence that adorned the place in the hall where Janice waited to walk up the aisle to be married.

The hall had filled to capacity long before the wedding was to begin. Three hundred people were invited, three hundred chairs were assembled, three hundred assembled chairs were occupied. Three hundred people sat with bated breath waiting for the beginning. Good or bad, for better or worse, the thing about extremity is that it clarifies. Life is not an endless repeat performance; it is precisely the opposite, however willfully blind we live our lives. Every moment of every day is new, fleeting, never to be repeated, and does not even happen if we miss it—that is, live it without our full attention. Even then, as we take in the fulsome holy moment, we cannot hold it, cannot keep it before our eyes, and only with deliberate intention can we infer proper meaning and commit to meaningful memory.

At five minutes to the hour our guest soloist was ready to sing. With James in his impeccable tuxedo playing the priceless antique grand piano, Marie Claire, in a long formal gown, hushed the excited crowd with her opening notes. "O Mio Babbino Caro" was the chosen opening aria and set the mood with just the right ingredients of beauty, solemnity, and high stakes emotion. Little did we know that we were about to be outdone.

Next up was the walk down the aisle to Janice's choice of recorded music. Long formal wear, divas, tuxedoes, and grand pianos have nothing on Aerosmith for moments of celebration and solemnity. It should be noted that we had not had time to absorb the music combination so we were as taken as the audience by the eclectic effect. All eyes were fixed on Janice and Eddy as they slowly made their way from far reaches to the front of the hall where long gown, tuxedo, diva, and grand piano lay dormant. And it must be said, Janice looked as alive as any human being ever was, while Eddy looked mostly happy and only a little bewildered. Memories and photos of Janice during the eternity of that two-minute stroll speak not to life as once lived but to life in perpetuity. It is why the crowd was singularly fixed on the walk and not the stationary pianist and soloist at the front. Still, while the crowd basked in the holy moment, I glanced over to James, who was not only watching but listening to Steve Tylor belt it out, with an expression that suggested less holy moment than *when will this moment ever end?* Actually, James was very gracious, the extent of his raised eyebrow merely suggesting that the music choices offered interesting contrast.

As Janice and Eddie walked down the aisle with Steven Tyler wailing *Don't want to miss a thing,* people looked at the couple with reverence, neither wanting nor willing to miss a thing. People had cancelled trips, abandoned family obligations, to attend and now stood in communion with the couple because we shared knowing and were unwilling to say otherwise. Janice, looking as good, rested, and healthy as she ever had in life, was going to die, and soon. "I Don't Want to Miss a Thing" was beautiful because we didn't miss a thing, we didn't deny a thing, and the thing that was going to happen, and soon, was outside and unable to affect this holy moment. Either denial or a rare glimpse into the indivisibility of love.

Waiting beside the grand piano was the woman who was going to marry the long overdue couple. Dawn Brown had been my boss before exiting the university to do, among other things, marry people. Primary among other things was working as a grief counsellor, which seemed an oddly fitting combo, particularly for this marriage. When Dawn's husband, Lawrence, had died far too young — the same year they had adopted a two-year-old boy from Jamaica — she became acutely aware of the need and importance of timely grief counselling. In more recent years, Dawn had moved from the intensity of grief counselling to the event of many emotions called marriage. (Reminds me of the three rings of marriage: the engagement *ring*, the wedding *ring*, and the suffe*ring*.)

Everyone had wanted to help out — as is our pathetic and noble way to assuage death — and Dawn was the first person I had called the evening we set upon our little scheme. She was perfect because the wedding/grief combo was what we all really needed, life being that Shakespearean interplay between comedy and tragedy, with tragedy mostly winning — well, depending on what you believe. That day, that night, comedy was front and centre (we're talking Janice after all) with tragedy always lurking on the periphery, but more to the point, everyone was looking at the bride in high comedic form.

After the ceremony and while we still had the great open hall, those who wanted to speak had their chance. All speeches were from colleagues, and in retrospect, we probably scared her family away. We didn't quite factor in that the world's loudest and most extreme extrovert might not have family members equally out there. For my part, I borrowed a short recording from a radio interview Janice had done in hospital a few days earlier. Hospitals are sombre places where death and disease are either happening or waiting with smug inevitability, so the happy-go-lucky mood of the office was tough to replicate. Janice didn't notice, even though the interviewer asked difficult questions about the toughness of life—that is, death. Janice answered without deflecting, and she laughed. And laughed. Long, loud, signature cackle, distinctively Janice.

With a ten-second repeating laugh spasm prelooped in my phone, I simply said, "I wanted to give you a sense of Janice without using words." I played her looped and loopy laugh into the microphone, and people laughed, a searing insight into the essence of Janice, an evocation of that short span between comedy and tragedy. We all knew we'd soon miss a thing called Janice. Just after the wedding I learned that a close friend had blurted out to Janice that she should use the laugh loop played at her wedding for her funeral. For most people, that would be an ouch moment that could never be recalled. Not Janice. She just laughed and said, "good idea."

The expectant crowd savoured every second of the wedding; I couldn't wait for it to end. The timing of the firemen arriving in their formal regalia was tricky for many reasons. The surprise would fall flat if they marched in before the wedding was over—or else it would be tragic and spectacular when Janice left Eddie at the altar and ran away with her four new lovers. I also didn't think they'd hang around long if we asked them to wait in the wings. Plus, there was that little detail of the fire truck they were going to arrive in, and for which we had no parking plan. People had been told to drive to the reception once the wedding was done. Still, we wanted them to stay to witness the big surprise, but milling about was going to be restricted in consideration of Janice's limited energy—so we thought.

The wedding ended, and the photographer ordered the bride, groom, and family to stand in choice locations for wedding photos. People prepared to leave, and I realized I was unprepared for managing the guests. I wanted people to stay, but I didn't want them to think I wanted them to stay. I wanted Janice's surprise to be complete. And then four strapping lads in full uniform carrying champagne and flowers appeared at the edge of the crowd waiting to be noticed. On Joycelyn's signal the four uniforms moved forward, parting the curious crowd, interrupting the family photography session and one bewildered bride. Janice glided towards the uniformed crew, less Cinderella with Prince Charming to the ballroom floor than shark to pool of unsuspecting fish.

Eddie looked like a deer in the headlight, but he knew what he had to do. My contact fireman had given Joycelyn the requested scruffy firefighting outfit, and she had immediately taken it to the nearby storage room as arranged. Eddie, Janice's husband of ten minutes, faded backwards and disappeared. With firemen in place, erect and formally attired, if anyone had asked about Eddie, Janice might have responded, "Eddie who?"

As Janice gloried and groped (well, bit of stretch, but not much) her four admirers, Amanda gave me the signal, and I played Bruce Springsteen's "Fire" from my phone over the sound system. At which precise moment, Eddie strutted out as fireman extraordinaire. Janice was so taken by her four formal firemen fantasy that at first she didn't notice. But as all eyes, and soon everyone's attention, went from the group of formal firemen to the rough and tumble informal fireman strutting his borrowed stuff, the object of Janice's desire shifted—possibly for the first time in their 23-year relationship—squarely on to Eddie. (Turns out it's not true that all eyes are on the bride at a wedding.) In that short distance between bride and groom, Eddie metamorphosed into swashbuckler, man of action, front cover of newest Harlequin romance, and was no longer an object of derision, Janice's sidekick, or mild-mannered Clark Kent.

They met in the middle of the hall—likely first time Janice ever met Eddie halfway—surrounded by a cheering crowd as Bruce wailed out "Fire," the highlight of their life, their love, their moment. (Makes you wonder why we bothered with the wedding part of the day.) Who knew that Eddie was going to be the exemplar of a central theme in this book regarding the singularity of each of life's moments? From the metaphoric backseat of a very long car, the hitherto predictable Eddie cruised around the room, a swaggering unknown figure with whom lay great mystery and a fetching sense of style. Twenty-three years in, and Eddie was reborn in Janice's eyes with his catwalk cruise. It's only over when there is no longer mystery.

We hadn't known it then, but the media had heard of and were covering the social and news event of the century. When Janice and Eddie met, they embraced and laughed, the moment captured for antiquity and for the front page of city newspapers the next day as the top story for the nation's capital that weekend. Something to revisit, often, in that non-sequential time thing I've conjured in my head by way of my heart. Illogical, nonsensical for sure, if not for the dangling detail of if not, what else?

It had been an exhausting first half of the wedding day, and we worried about Janice's fatigue. Before the firemen could leave there were multiple photos taken outdoors in front of the fire truck with the group surrounding a glowing Janice. They left and left us with the distinct impression that this little volunteer venture was unlike whatever number of assignments they had ever agreed to in the past. Good for them, bewilderment aside. At the reception, Janice didn't just mingle with her "peeps"; she seemed to be in six places at the same time, sort of a benign Hurricane Janice flailing across the landscape.

Eddie, now out of his testosterone firefighting outfit, reverted to his former self—though a decidedly happier version—and gratefully faded behind Janice's commanding presence. She talked, she danced, she laughed, all the while defying physical world confinement to time and place, and even as the restaurant was closing and the last of the last of the guests said goodbye for the umpteenth time, adding that it was the best wedding they had ever attended, Janice continued as a whirling dervish without the slightest hint of fatigue. It wasn't that she was healed. It had been her day, and she hadn't wanted to miss a thing. She hadn't miss a thing; she was the thing.

To this day, people who attended Janice and Eddie's wedding will stop and compare their impressions of the magic that was. And the impressions that were,

were eerily similar. Twenty-three years into their relationship the newlyweds were gracious and grateful, and we who had planned it felt some small sense of not accomplishment but relief for having been, if nothing else, a bit less useless about Janice's illness. The glow never left Janice, but her health worsened, and we reverted to our state of uselessness. We briefly wondered if the firemen's sense of volunteer duty extended to agreeing to marrying Janice, one after the other, each wedding bigger and better, but no, not fair to Eddie, so we reluctantly had to admit that there was nothing we could do.

God love her, as she worsened, she continued to talk, not about getting better, since she knew otherwise, but about coming back to work. We had not filled Janice's job (good luck filling Janice's vacated space) and had instead opted to use young people part-time piecemeal, out of loyalty and to assuage her unrealistic fear that she could be replaced and realistic fear that she would soon miss everything.

She was stable until the end of August. We kept in touch, she was on our minds, but work, family, conferences, holidays—before we knew it, our short northern summer, less seasonal than fleeting, was almost over. None of us would have admitted it, but at some level we all thought that we could pick up with Janice in September where we had left off in June. We humans do this and miss most of everything.

The combination of life-sustaining drugs and time served inside a hospital during our exquisitely short summer stripped Janice of her vitality. She was pale and pasty, her skin as white as her regrown hair. Heavy steroid use caused her to look bloated, giving her face an unnaturally round cartoonish look that contrasted with the look of young tanned and rested visitors who felt dread for Janice even as their eyes were drawn to the window, to the outside world that they would exit back into as soon as possible. Still, and still being Janice, she momentarily reversed the ravages of cancer—cancer drugs that only work when they are nearly killing the cancer patient—and the depressive monotony of hospital life with spontaneous laughter and a few well-placed insulting barbs designed to say *I love you* in response to the forlorn looks on our faces. In short, she assuaged our guilt and made us feel better. Which wasn't the direction that relief was supposed to flow in, in our well-intended useless minds.

Our short visits were not a problem—Janice was incapable of grievances, and she tired easily. Frequent visits were best; besides, Eddie and Janice's two adult children, Scott and Tammy, by a first marriage, kept vigilance so she was never alone. Many people came, the tone always fun, frivolous, gossipy, with much slagging and the like. Still, for someone who didn't want to miss a thing, possibly something was missing. Dr. John, our resident psychologist, wanted to visit. Janice considered John one of her peeps, so he would be welcomed. John had lost a son in the recent past and was a practising Buddhist, so his take on Janice's situation was a bit different than that of her other visitors.

After two years of cheerfully submitting to every sickening and invasive procedure, she had just been told that the end was near. Perhaps a couple weeks.

John and I talked and wondered if, even as fun and frivolity continued, Janice might want to make room for real discussion, an acknowledgement of death. John's well-informed Buddhist thought was that one can have a good death by embracing two simple concepts. The first concept is to approach death with an open heart, which sounded beautiful for both its simplicity and its impossibly. But I am an angst-ridden Catholic and not a converted, relaxed Buddhist, so no credibility there. Still, we agreed that if ever there was a human soul who could approach death with a wide and open, gaping open, heart, it was Janice. First concept, easy.

The second concept is to approach death without fear. People not staring death in the eye often talk abstractly about facing it easily, fearlessly, heroically even, but few of us without the mind of a saint can pull it off. Faith in an afterlife, belief that there is something for each of us after bearing the trifecta of pain and loss and death, is tough enough to declare, tougher still to fully believe, toughest yet to embrace. This life, much as we live illusion, is what we know, and it is hard to fully know that life after death has a life. People who experience the radiant white light of a near-death experience offer comfort, but when looking at a dead body we all understand that the body that lived and moved and loved hours earlier is not resting, is not asleep, is dead. We just know. Since we all share knowledge of the certainty of not just death but our own imminent death, isn't conversation with someone who is dying an opportunity to lay bare our common humanity, to listen and hear the inarticulate speech of their departing heart? Knowing death without knowing how to talk to people about death can isolate a dying person in a way that the distracted living often overlook.

Between the hordes of visiting frivolity, John and I slipped in to see Janice, and I encouraged him to give Janice permission to talk about death if she was so inclined. After the requisite number of hugs and jokes, John asked if he could say something. As he explained the concept of approaching death with an open heart, I chimed in with my version of how Janice had pulled that off spectacularly during her two-year ordeal. Janice didn't respond, perhaps from denial, thoughts too painful for words — we didn't know. John paused and then continued with the second concept. This time Janice became animated and responded with emphasis, "That's me! I'm not afraid!" And the thing is, she wasn't, and as the weeks ticked down from days to hours, she remained fearless. She just wasn't afraid.

Janice died in September. She lived longer than any of her many doctors, the experts, had predicted, had expected. Which shouldn't be a surprise really. They deal in life, not death, and death is more than the cessation of life. Their analysis had been limited to tests and textbooks and her reaction to procedures and treatments. They had not attended her wedding and were not privy to the song she had selected to walk down the aisle.

In her last days, Janice was in pain, was heavy sedated, was in and out of a coma and, increasingly, mostly in. My last visit was in the late afternoon of the day before she died. The days of late August into September had been an unbroken succession of clear bright skies. Such weather in Canada is bittersweet as it migrates from perfection to perdition. For Canadians, summer is nine parts anticipation followed by one part regret. Merely weeks after lazy summer days comes the fading of heat and light for the encroachment of dark and cold that is to be our winter of discontent. Winter never seems to anticipate summer and, once descended, seems only to be what it is. I suppose an analogy to faith lurks here, for however brutal, cold, and dark the season, we are challenged to believe that spring will come.

Walking from my car, I was reluctant to surrender outside perfection for hospital imperfection, radiant open air for suffocating indoor sterility. Janice had always wanted to escape Canadian winter oppression for the open air of Hawaii. Her intention had always been stifled by crass finances so remained unrealized, as so much did in her life. The previous year, Janice's daughter had started a collection to fulfill her bucket list, which we gladly contributed to in the spirit of doing something. But then we found out that crass finances were no longer the problem, because insurance would not cover out-of-country travel, and Janice could not risk needing medical treatment. Without protest she let Hawaii slip away, as had become the reality of her life. Not a big deal for the outward Janice; she simply made a transfer from her bucket list to her F-it list. In addition to ribald genius, Janice never lost her happy fatalism.

I know this is what she would have said, but I never actually got the chance to ask her. Even in slow motion, things move fast. On that last afternoon, I was glad that only Janice and Eddie were in the room. Janice was unconscious, was not expected to gain consciousness, should have been dead, we were reminded. Eddie was low-key and quiet, his eternal vigilance flattening his personality with an unnatural ennui. I stood by her bedside like an a**e, stroking her hand, talking nonsense, still unused to a Janice who did not respond to everything and anything I said. Eddie spoke once in a while, whenever I ran out of nonsense, always sweetly, always tenderly, always—even in consideration of firemen in her life—with love.

It was time to leave, this time with finality. I wasn't going to linger. Janice and I had a great relationship, but I was far from the most important person coming to say goodbye. Besides, though still alive, she was gone to awareness of her life and all of us in it.

I consciously said to myself, *Take one last look, pause, lift your hand off her arm, turn, and leave.* I walked to the foot of the bed, made it to the doorway, and heard Eddie exclaim, "Would you look at that!" I turned around, first seeing Eddie's expression of amazement, and then Janice, with what can only be described as her biggest, most radiant smile, verging on her world-altering laugh. I stood still, Eddie rose to his feet, and Janice's smile held, just as it had been, surely one of the world's most memorable events, a visible manifestation of the essential fact of life, evident to all of us all the time if only we would notice: love is, and remains, even in our despair. I could interpret Janice's smile as a revelation and parting gift or else insignificant wonky brain function as it atrophied from dysfunction to non-function. No mystery what my interpretation is. Janice knew I didn't want to miss a thing so gave me a thing to miss, which I gratefully still do.

Janice didn't exit easily; not wanting to miss a thing cost her. She painfully groaned and thrashed all night and into the next day without relief. Eddie was magnificent, talking, soothing her, telling her she could go, and if she could have responded she might have answered, "I know, dummy, but then I'd miss a thing or two, wouldn't I?"

A large group was uncomfortably gathered mostly outside her room on that last day, listening uselessly to Janice's uneasy exit, her inability or unwillingness to let go. Her fight was so unexpectedly ferocious that when the moment finally came, the primary spontaneous emotion was more relief than grief. Who knew Janice would exit like Raging Bull fighting for the title, punch-drunk and senseless, resisting until the very end? God love her.

The question is this: Is Janice missing a thing? Lurking outside of conventional science and logic is faith, but like Rodney Dangerfield, it doesn't get much respect. (Okay, so weird analogy, but Janice would like it, so it remains as written.) Modern nihilists disparage but do not answer the question, or else offer explanations that are unintelligible, less explanation than explaining away what cannot be answered in material-world language. To which I again ask the squarest, most archaic, and un-coolest question of all time: If not, what else? What explains the inexplicable?

These moments, Janice's laugh, my stories, will not fully explain or fulfill but are closer, have to be closer, to truth than the cosmology of multiverses, universes from nothing, and the biology of cells that live and are no more, all as products of the infinitesimal impossibility, 'Cause *it's what nothingness does over infinite time and space, don't ya know?* If my answer leaves doubt, good, for that is the nature of a living faith while we live. Materialism and modernity tag-team denial of death—not that it happens, but that it could possibly have meaning. Maybe Aerosmith should write a song for the era called "You Won't Miss a Thing 'Cause Death Doesn't Mean a Thing." Or maybe we should put our faith in Sir Conan Doyle's Sherlock Holmes, whose most famous sleuthing quote is as follows: "Once you eliminate the impossible, whatever remains, no matter how improbable, must be truth." Faith is what we suspect, hope for, or know beneath all the reasons not to believe.

As far as I could tell, Janice wasn't particularly concerned about faith, either having it or not. She didn't sweat the logic, the science, the prevailing creeping atheist worldview, possibly because there is nothing funny in any of their arguments. But whether conscious or not, angst-ridden or not, Janice had enough of the *stuff*— that is, the internal logic of faith—not to be afraid when the grim reaper stood by her bedside. Whether like Dr. John, who doesn't articulate reasons for having faith for what he knows (knowledge beyond language, and consequently faith of the highest order) or something else we cannot access but exists nonetheless, the phenomenology of Janice's life, laugh, and substantive speech is a rarely accomplished articulation of the inexplicable heart, and that, my friends, is enough.

Reasons not to believe are generally not what we know (except for that know-it-all Dr. John) but rather what seeps in through the vacuum of denial. Post-religion post-faith modernity is a Faustian selling of the soul wherein the fiction that *life is but a dream* subverts troubling thoughts of inevitable death, for a finite time. But the troubling fact of life is that death, stark and unnuanced, and for all we deny, visits upon us without Richard Dawkins sitting by our bedside holding our hand with reassuring words about material meaning after the cessation of cellular function. The Faustian bargain must be repaid and comes with the deeply repressed revelation that physical death is merely the concluding detail to a forfeited spiritual life.

Chapter Nine

SUPERMEN

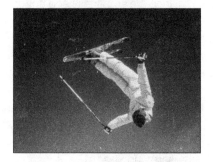

"Superman never made any money
And sometimes I despair
The world will never see another man like him."
"Superman's Song," from the *Ghost That Haunts Me* album,
Crash Test Dummies (1991)

I remember when I was a kid hearing that there are not hundreds or thousands but millions of stars up above the sky. And when I learned that there is a bigger number than millions, I was staggered by the fact that there are more likely billions of stars. Same for when I learned that even billions actually has an exponentially greater number called trillions. (UCSB ScienceLine estimates there are one billion trillion stars in the universe or, for laymen dummies like me, an amount approximating the number of grains of sand on all the beaches on the entire earth.) Trillions of stars, each with a physical mass much bigger than Earth, twinkling out at night as we wee humans watch from a bedroom window below. And I wondered, How can God make more stars within the singularity of expanding space than we can even begin to mentally grasp? Silly question, but I wanted to know, though I might reframe the question today as What are the limits to the physical universe? And being the pain that I am, that question naturally leads to this: What precisely is our speck of humanity doing in the far outreaches of darkness and mostly nothingness punctuated by rare clumps of meaningless matter?

A familiar answer: meaning is what you make of it. But with nihilism in full bloom, that answer seems a tad disingenuous. Whether or not one describes oneself as having or not having faith, we all hang our hats on, have faith in, something, not nothing, even if our something adds up to nothing. Materialism rules, therefore there is no transcendent meaning, so you get to spend your life extracting meaning from material-world things. Make sense? I'm not being cynical. We are creatures of pathos and heroism, intention and contradiction; it is how we get from one minute to the next. Not thinking about this does not negate framing our life within a multiplicity of distractions. We do not exist in a vacuum—though looking into space it comes mighty close—so we conjure up, invest in, something to grasp, to make real, to give us context to counterbalance the emptiness and entropy of a universe of a size and expanding at a rate that is impossible to comprehend. There is much that we humans understand but cannot comprehend.

We are complacent and unthinking in the age of anxiety, the former being the reason for the later. We embrace distraction into an unexamined life; then we ignore the consequences. Still, the examined life is not all cerebral; the practice of faith, not only spiritual. A life well lived may be equal parts examined and example.

From first memory, Mike Nemesvary lived for adventure, sport, and motion. Fully 35 years after he became a quadriplegic—though he is transformed, fully adapted, and matured—the same applies. Mike is incapable of significant motion below the neck, yet lives for motion, both literally and figuratively, without a hint of contradiction. Mike had a cataclysmic accident from which few of us could recover. In a single moment, he lost most of the world-class physicality that had defined his life. Adapting to a world where all has been lost defies logic.

By his own admission, Mike was cocky, confident, a driven and talented athlete with plans for glory and every reason to believe that his expectations would be realized. Great athletes do not tend to have the disposition of Mahatma Gandhi. The list of Mike's early accomplishments is long, so highlights will have to suffice. In 1970, he won the Ontario junior championship for lacrosse before switching to skiing as his main sport. During the next few years, he was the Canadian junior champion in aerials, moguls, ballet, and overall. Between 1976 and 1980, Mike was the Canadian champion in all categories of freestyle skiing before sliding onto the world stage as an adult and winning Italian, French, British, and world freestyle championships. Somehow between Canadian slopes and the world stage, Mike won the Canadian trampoline championship, an ominous foreshadowing.

At the beginning of the new decade, Mike is verging on becoming an international sports celebrity; he is tall, good-looking, exceptionally accomplished for one so young; he has friends and admirers, particularly women, whom he is particularly interested in. Not only does his athletic prowess make him a hero; he is making a name for himself commercially. You can still see Mike at his prime in opening skiing scenes from the 1985 James Bond film *A View to a Kill*. Marvel at the poetry in motion while trying to disregard the cheesy plot. Dangerous descents, dramatic stunts, raw power, but still graceful, elegant, and in complete control. That is Mike Nemesvary, for whom the cliché actually and metaphorically applied: in skiing and in life, he was on top of the world.

Though Mike grew up in Canada, he was born in Glasgow, Scotland, has dual citizenship, and decided to represent Great Britain. He lives in a quaint cottage with a nice girlfriend so he can blister around the countryside in his sports car (what else?). On a sunny off-season Saturday afternoon in May he gets together with his girlfriend and friends for beer and steaks. Pleasant, regular social routine. Someone suggests they try out Mike's trampoline that he uses to train during the off-season. It is stored at a friend's nearby farm, so the group organizes themselves to drive over. Once the trampoline is set up, his friends go first, and then it is Mike's turn.

Even off-season, even among friends, even participating in an activity that is not his competitive sport, he is competitive. Mike has not been on a trampoline since before winter, but his friends' performances have been unimpressive, and, well, Mike is a self-described show-off. He is rusty but does some maneuvers 14 feet into the air, and then ups the height and level of difficulty by doing a triple backwards somersault on skies, but loses his orientation to the ground, hits the trampoline completely out of control and on the back of his neck. Suffice to say, the reality of *completely out of control* has entered Mike's life and is to be his daily, hourly reality for the rest of his life. Though it is a self-described freak accident, Mike Nemesvary, age 24, is laid bare to the brute force inevitability of life in the material world.

Mike lay fully awake, fully aware, but without feeling. He was scared but did not panic. He felt a warm sensation in his limbs, a mild precursor to the unfeeling horror that was to be his life. If physical sensation were the lifeblood of his soul, he could feel it leave his body, and for the past 35 years he has experienced in every second of every day its absolute absence.

An ambulance was called, arriving 15 minutes later. He was taken to a local hospital where a doctor stuck pins into his limbs and asked if he could feel anything. After he responded negatively, an invasive tube was stuck down his throat to take over the function of breathing that Mike was quickly losing. The tube was terribly intrusive, and he was heavily medicated and in and out of consciousness as he was transferred by ambulance to the Stanmore Hospital due to the complexity of his case. After the necessary surgery to stabilize his neck, he was then completely unconscious for two days. The ten-hour operation performed by a neurosurgeon involved cutting off a piece of shin bone and fusing it to the broken vertebrae in his neck. Mike was then screwed, literally, through the head, into traction, complete immobility, completely out of control. Mike is no longer an athlete, master of motion, movie phenomenon, admired man about town; he is a high-level C 4–5, complete break to spinal column, quadriplegic. His life ends as he sleeps; his new life begins, such as it will be, the moment he awakens.

Upon waking, Mike is only able to move his eyes. His head and neck are held in traction, with metal pegs driven into his skull bone. A ventilation and gastric tube has been inserted down his throat. He cannot move; he cannot breathe on his own; he cannot eat; he cannot speak. An errant fly lands on his nose and slowly murders by a thousand itches. Less pain than frustration, though torture nonetheless. He tries to communicate with his eyes, an exercise—ironic use of the word—in frustration that almost makes the fly on his nose seem delightful.

Disturbing as these restrictions were, there was worse, far worse. Mike's lung collapsed, and he was given a highly invasive bronchoscopy. A long tube was inserted down his throat and into the collapsed lung so doctors could observe the problem and attempt to apply suction lines. The procedure requires that the patient be conscious throughout in order that he not swallow his tongue. The procedure, taking a full 45 minutes, was hell, was worse than water boarding, longer, more painful, inducing the absolute panic of drowning without foreknowledge of outcome. Just writing the sentence makes me claustrophobic. I want to give thanks and be grateful even as I feel a stranglehold of panic.

The news of Mike Nemesvary's accident is a big story in Britain and internationally. The high flyer has been grounded, the burning star extinguished; the spectacular super nova explosion is *the* news story for that weekend in May and beyond, with all its titillating detail, excitement, and lurking schadenfreude that is attendant upon every human tragedy. Much of celebrity fascination has this schadenfreudian caring—that is, the secret delight in another's misfortune, the curled lip that belies the words of concern. Even the mighty fall and, for some, weirdly, the details help assuage the meaningless of their little lives. Headlines know their audience. "Triumph and Tragedy of Bond Star," June 18, 1985, in the *Daily Express*, by Peter Hardy: "Four weeks ago, British ski champion Mike Nemesvary had the world, if not always at his feet, at least spinning beneath him. The 24-year old ranked fourth in the world of freestyle skiing, held the Canadian, British, and European titles, and looked forward to a possible gold in the 1988 Winter Olympics." Weeks after his accident (long by media standards), Mike's story still gets some coverage because of his recent accomplishments, medal potential, and the sad juxtaposition of dreams lost and nightmares found.

Even after the story has faded, the tabloids see an opportunity to resurrect it in the name of love. A photo of Mike and his girlfriend (punctuated by the beauty of youth and the tell-tale features of 1980s fashion) frame the front page with bold headlines: "One Woman's Very Special Love: A Tragedy Strikes Down Her Boyfriend but Their Love Goes On"; that is, until she goes away, as was always most likely. Still, for that one cover shot and sensational headline, readers and sensation seekers suspended what was most likely for what we liked. And the great unwashed public likes or even loves enduring love, whether or not it is backed up by truth. The tabloid cover further titillates: "In an exclusive interview CHAT magazine finds out how love has helped the brave 25-year-old fight back." If only the effort to fight back could be contained by a moment in time, gloriously depicted by youth, beauty, and bravery. Thirty-five years on, Mike contends with quadriplegia, the effort of each measured day not reflected in that tabloid photo, including or especially the 1980s styles that he has moved on from. Girlfriend a distant memory, youth and beauty equally removed, only the daily grind, that non-tabloid hard-won scraping of effort over time continuing in muted, unspectacular fashion. To the world, the sensation of May 18, 1985, has been relegated to yesterday's news.

Still, for a limited time, friends, family, and newly acquired famous people flocked to Mike's bedside—including Princess Diana—to give what comfort and support were possible. Photos of Mike in bed after injury, early in rehab, and the first time in his wheelchair show him smiling. I haven't seen any photos of Mike without a smile or with an expression that might capture what he actually was feeling and how he might have assessed his future adjusting to the incomprehensible. Curiously, later photos and Mike's written recollections of that time similarly do not betray his feelings, even as he divulges his thoughts. His reflections on the cataclysm are about purpose, the glow of drive from the embers of a lost life, all business, no emotion, impersonally narrated in the third person.

> His first order of business was to move into an accessible cottage, develop a relationship, independently drive a modified sports car and complete the documentary *Same Games—Different Rules* (Interface Productions/S.P.A. Ltd./Aspect Films). While still undergoing rehabilitation, he had the unique opportunity to go "sit-skiing" in Switzerland just five months following his accident which positively changed his outlook on life and vowed to reinvent his life by continuing to live an active lifestyle which included swimming, weight lifting, water skiing, scuba diving and adventure seeking.

A qualifying *by the way* is appropriate here. No one goes "sit-skiing" five months after sustaining a complete C4–5 broken spinal column. It is not possible, except for the fact that Mike did just that. Certainly not on the advice of his doctors, and without doubt against the advice of said doctors. There was huge risk, and even the fragile spinal column—with a bone graft from a distant shin—might not have fully stabilized. Denial? Perhaps, but really another word is needed for someone who knows the risks and proceeds fully, enthusiastically, and without reservation for no other reason than that it is what he must do. Mike could endure the unendurable of spinal cord injury; Mike could not endure limiting risky behaviour due to spinal cord injury. It is his purpose, and Mike's life depends on doing everything with purpose. Not a death wish so much as a requirement for life. Move or die, even if you can't move.

Which raises the question, Where does such drive—and under impossible circumstances—come from? Mike consciously chose to remake himself using the tools of strength of character and competitiveness for which he was famous pre-accident. He applied his pre-accident resolve to new circumstances, so *denial* is not the defining word. Mike was painfully aware that he was not going to ski as he used to, but he was determined to proceed without compromise and do what no quadriplegic has ever done. Given the devastation that high-level spinal cord injury is, this resolve is fairly astonishing. The rehab gig is designed to eventually allow patients to transfer from a bed into a wheelchair and does not include getting from a wheelchair into a sit-ski contraption to launch down Alpine mountains.

To expand upon the previous paragraph's question: Is Mike's drive an example of intention that is *the* distinguishing feature of life and the unfolding of our universe—the evidence of which is everywhere at all times these 13.7 billion years and counting—or is it just part of arbitrary atoms and cells naturally and unintentionally selecting towards meaningless arbitrary outcomes? If the latter seems silly, Mike's inexplicable drive only becomes explicable when considered as one human example of ever-unfolding pervasive universal intention. Overblown as this may seem, existence does come down to either shards of intention and design or fantastically complex and statistically impossible nothingness. I puzzle over the purpose people have who have no faith, who actively embrace the nothingness of existence throughout their lives. Mike likely wasn't thinking this as he catapulted off a mountain, and yet there are beacons of faith in action that outrank all the theory in the world. Maybe action figures are heroes for a reason.

Mike decides, and then he actually does it—all of it. There will be low or no glory, no or fewer women, hero worship replaced by occasional admiration; the uphill battle will be much tougher than the downhill slide, and gravity will never again seem to be working in his favour. But if nothing else, he is not immobilized by physical inertia; he makes what choices he can, the only choices left to a creature of intention and action.

Mike's life motto might be a variation on the New Hampshire licence plate: Live exceptional or die. Parenthetically, I wrote the last sentence and then boarded a plane in warm Cato, Cuba, to go back home to ice and snow. I uncharacteristically watched a romance called *I Before You*, about a handsome, rich, and athletic young man who becomes a quadriplegic. The narrative arch has to do with his desperation to die coupled with the fact that he meets a beautiful, poor, lower class girl (yes, it is British), and they—seemingly against the odds, but actually quite inevitably—fall in love. The young man has a potential suicide plan that involves going to an expensive Swiss clinic. Apart from my misgivings about romantic films in general and about this one in particular, the film becomes rather charming. We are moved along, caught up in the relationship, and fully convinced that immobile Prince Charming will come to his senses, become inspiring, and, with his blossoming Cinderella, choose life.

But he doesn't. The audience is confronted by the great reversal—far more common in film today, often in contravention of preceding narrative progression and common sense. For six months after injury he despaired of his life and came to an agreement with his parents. If after one full year he still wished to end his life, they would support him. At this point he has not met the love of his life, and of course the next six months feature the magic of that relationship with the poor girl convincing the rich guy that his life is worth living. He seems to become happy, seems to have come around to both life and, most important, his life with her. We who are watching have fallen in love with her, so how can he say no? The film ends with the protagonist choosing "I before you," as the title foretold, which turns out to be choosing suicide. We end up feeling both unsettled and a little sheepish for not guessing the outcome based on the title. Or maybe my lack of romantic film consumption just made me gullible.

In the film, Will had claimed that life was not possible for someone who had been as active as he had been pre-accident. I guess we're not supposed to blame Will for his decision—and yet us hopeless romantics and the girl he left behind were manipulated into believing he was going to choose "you" before "I." It occurred to me that suicide, rather than either of the couple, was given the romantic lead, even though the choice of suicide is easier than the choice to live. The thing about Mike that is central to his life is this: the golden boy for whom life was but a dream was spectacularly unprepared for the real hardship that had become his life. Sure, winning athletic contests takes fortitude, but contests end, and we are left with life and all its tragic complexity and hardship and the slow drip of time once the friends, media, and photo seekers have all gone home. Mike was dealt cruel cards, his life more nightmare than dream, and he has been called on to make difficult choices with courage ever since. And hard as this verdict is, Mike compounded this tough choice scenario by choosing, always, at all turns, the toughest road.

Mike's logic—equal parts determination and contradiction—was to superimpose the freedom and perpetual motion of his old life onto his new life as a quadriplegic. Consistent with his athletic accomplishments pre-accident, Mike chose to extend boundaries—that is, motion without mobility. A couple of selective examples. In 1987, Mike chose a sporting goal—to break the toboggan land speed record. This would be unadvisable motion for a quadriplegic attempting to break a record set by another quadriplegic, but no, Mike had his sights set on the land speed record for *all* humans, all time. Interviewed before the attempt, he said, "I need something, an athletic goal. I've still got something inside me that tells me I'm a sportsman." Reminds me of a line from "The Taxi," an iconic Harry Chaplin song: "I've got something inside me to drive a princess blind." Though not a popular notion in material-world thinking, the *something inside me,* the something inside Mike, does not go away easily, is not a material-world thing to lose. Those who risk and lose tend to become risk adverse. Not Mike. If risk got him into this situation, it was bloody well going to get him out. As for the insanely dangerous land speed attempt, it didn't succeed; Mike didn't accept it not succeeding so started planning for another attempt.

In 1992, Mike decided to go to the Winter Olympics in Albertville, France. Mike was not wired to be a spectator, and these were *the* Olympics where he had planned to stand on the podium. An Olympic medal had been a realistic goal. However, best laid plans can go awry and be supplanted by the *but for the grace of God* world that we inhabit, in which a guarantee of chaos is to tell God your plans. Mike made another plan. To achieve his new athletic goal, to break the toboggan land speed record (a plan now called The Sled Project), he realized that he needed a sponsor. What better place to meet a sporting sponsor than at the Olympics?

A quadriplegic travelling to the Olympics in winter, planning to do what Mike intended to do, at a time when the world was not much concerned with accessibility, was going to be challenged. If Mike had allowed for advice (which he did not) he would have certainly been advised not to go even if he had the support to pull it off (which he did not). So, there he is, flying with his clothes, equipment, and all the supplies he will need for his care that will not be available at the Olympics, as well as a forty-pound sled, a helmet, and a selection of splints needed to support his paralyzed hands and arms. Why take a sled to the Olympics, where certain restrictions apply, even before considering how the heck to transport the thing to the site? Mike says the idea was that the sled would allow him to "to get up and down the mountain and see the events close up."

Mike flies by himself to Geneva, Switzerland, and meets his good British friend Paul, and they drive six hours to be as close to the Olympic site as they can get, which isn't close. Mike has never been deterred by challenging logistics. He manages to watch a number of events close up, sees friends and former competitors winning medals, realizing dreams, feeling something inside to drive a princess blind. Mike won 18 World Cup competitions and more than 40 international titles before injury at an age far before his prime. Most of the winners are less accomplished than Mike, and two years later in Lillehammer, Norway, as his sport evolves from demonstration into full Olympic status, fellow competitor Sonny Schonbichler wins the much coveted first gold medal in aerials, Mike's specialty. During all his years of competition, Sonny had never won a World Cup event, but as happens in sport, he peaked at the exact right time (or else got lucky), and history records that he is the first aerials gold medalist. Sonny won, but Mike coulda been a contenda.

Shoulda actually, but life is not like that. Life is not fair, does not yield to our expectations, is an indifferent lover, though it is possible that we are looking for love in all the wrong places. Mike thinks and talks about these lost fragments, but he is not a creature of resentment. And though it was with far less glory, little fanfare, and a heap of aggravation and grief, it is no cliché to say that what he has achieved since his competitive ski days is beyond peaking at the right moment for a World Cup title that not does transform, uplift, or contribute to humanity. Without joining the rarified club of Olympic gold medalists, Mike soared to a singular less well-known place in history, transcending immobility and physical constraints, even if most of his life is swallowed up in the minutia of material-world limitations.

Mike goes into a funk watching and not doing at the Albertville Olympics. He had brought a sled to be able to move and frankly to draw attention to himself in an attempt to raise sponsorship funds for his coming toboggan speed record. But he needs more. The way out of funk is focus. Mike—gregarious in the extreme—meets a Belgian guy named Pym who interests him in the concept of parapenting. Parapenting is hand gliding for skiers and can be done solo or with a partner, the latter making possible Mike's participation as a player, the prerequisite for whatever he undertakes. No passive couch-surfing for this guy. In his newly acquired life, he has to rely on people in a way that is never easy. Still, dependence caveat aside, he has plans for doing, completing, goals no other quadriplegic has ever attempted, restrictions be dammed.

Good thing Mike has brought his sled, though it is far from certain how it and he will fly. Still, you can't make an omelette without breaking a few legs, and since Mike can't feel his legs, there's no risk, right? It is a logistical nightmare to get Mike and his sled up the mountain and on site for a parapenting attempt. The earnest Belgian has been making elaborate adjustments, but no one knows if the attempt to fly will or can work. It is another logistical challenge to get Mike into place, into his sled, strapped into a four-point rally harness, legs secured and arm splints adjusted so that he can steer the levers attached to skis.

The first attempt is just about ready, and Mike is clear that he is willing to risk life and unfeeling limb in the pursuit of sporting glory. Several attempts result in several needed adjustments to equipment and logistical regroupings. Finally, adjustments and logistics are relegated to the rear-view mirror, Mike and the Belgian soar off the mountain, and they actually fly, not as easily as Mike once flew on skies, but he is a player again, he has accomplished something no quadriplegic has ever done, immobility has been vanquished, and history has been made for the eternity of about ten minutes.

While the preceding is true, it is also true that while Mike and the Belgian were soaring through the air they very nearly soared to their death. The parapenting pair and Mike's sled were too heavy, flying so low they almost scraped into a deadly mountain crevasse at high speed, barely recovering enough to land without death or injury. Being interviewed at the time and recounting the adventure since then, Mike has talked about the euphoria of flight and the freedom of movement. Only recently did he mention the near-death aspect to that experience, including the screams from the generous Belgian, who did not share Mike's willingness to risk life or limb, and in particular his feeling limbs.

If participation in sporting activities was foremost in Mike's war against immobility, reclaiming the freedom to drive was a close second. First problem: the right vehicle cost tons of money. Second problem: modifications to vehicles in the 1980s were not very good. I didn't know Mike then, but I remember Paul Menton's van—a constant source of frustration for the days, weeks, decades spent in the garage. And then out of tragedy came opportunity.

When I was an orderly in the early 1980s few of our young traumatized patients were female. Males are greater risk takers—that is, the type of risks parents would agree are unadvisable. But not always. Elaine Wolfe ended up on the spinal cord unit, a quadriplegic at age 18 due to a diving accident, wide-eyed with shock and bewilderment. No description can adequately do justice to her innocence, trapped in that place, at that time facing a life she could not imagine. But the reality of life is that we must often endure what we cannot imagine, the reality made harsher by the tender age it can visit upon its stupefied survivors. Exacerbating the juxtaposition between unimaginable and reality was that she had radiant beauty but had been co-opted into a world antithetical to things beautiful. It should be noted that Elaine did find beauty in life, in time. She, the youngest of seven girls, contributed to the universal evocation of beauty and had two daughters of her own.

Parents never really recover from the disruption to how life was supposed to unfold for their kid. A father's sense of failure to protect is devastating after a cataclysmic preventable accident. Elaine's father, Cliff, was an engineer and channeled his sense of bewilderment into problem solving. Among many other innovations he developed, Cliff made more than 100 Elaine Anne Lift Systems to assist people with spinal cord injury to get into and out of their own vehicles without assistance. Meanwhile, Mike was frustrated by driving modifications to his vehicles until he met Cliff Wolfe, whose problem-solving channeling had evolved into a thriving business. Mike was not a fan of mechanical breakdowns, but he really liked to drive. As always, he had plans.

In the spirit of always pursuing exceptionalism and wanting to always surpass his previous foray into over-the-top exceptionalism, Mike decided to drive around the world. He has never said so, but I think Mike absolutely loved to present over-the-top challenges as everyday innocuous activities. He was the natural pre-Nike precursor to *Just Do It,* making him refreshingly antithetical to the modern world. Virtue-signallers have forgotten the truth of the cliché that *actions speak louder than words.*

Once an idea entered his head, Mike had to see it through, though realizing his thought of driving around the world would take considerable time and logistical summersaulting. The Round the World Challenge took three years to plan, during which time Mike's logistical genius was on full display. First order of business was selling the concept, then in the glow of common purpose, he convinced people to volunteer the work required to move the project along. No precedent, limited resources, many barriers, and yet his drive to drive soon had both life and mobility. Mike was a bit like Tom Sawyer, who glamourized the concept of fence painting so that neighbourhood kids paid for the privilege of doing his work.

In fairness, for all the free labour he was able to galvanize and extract for any of his projects, no one worked harder than Mike. He chaired all Round the World Challenge meetings, oversaw all details, directed the many moving parts, and even managed to get the thing launched to much fanfare and media attention on Parliament Hill, on March 20, 2001, with Prime Minister Jean Chretien coming out to send off his good friend Mike Nemesvary in his customized truck. Fellow writer and long-time friend Rick Taylor and I came out to the send-off, and we noticed that Mike never relinquished being the centre of attention, with the prime minister relegated to a supporting role. Good for you, I thought then, and think the same today. Mike always has had an easy best pal's effect on princesses, prime ministers, famous Hollywood types, and paupers. And at the bottom of the list, me.

I disappointed Mike and did not volunteer over half a year of my life for the challenge. He understood that the risk of losing my wife, kids, and job was the reason, but this was just not a fully acceptable reason to a man possessed. Still, we remained friends, and I followed the challenge as best I could from my conventional stationary world. And, no surprise, but rather fantastically, he completed the whole bloody drive around the world, replete with a couple dozen unanticipated disasters, challenges, and showstoppers that would have felled most people—well, anyone who was not Mike. That would be seven months, 21 countries, and more than 40,000 kilometres of tough roads, inhospitable weather, and unsavoury politics to contend with. Not only that, without the media attention of Rick Hansen's Man in Motion Tour years earlier, Mike raised $1.5 million for spinal cord research, which fuelled bigger plans, for which he has established precedence.

In addition to his insatiable desire for adventure, Mike raises awareness about barriers that people with disabilities face and accomplishments that the same are still capable of achieving. And nothing creates awareness better than raising money. Within a year of his accident—just after he managed to figure out a way to ski again—he and an influential friend decided to create a charity to help other spinal cord injured people recover some semblance of their former active life (the idea being that most mortals do not have Mike's superhuman drive and might need a figurative and supportive push). With Barbara Broccoli (renowned producer of the James Bond film franchise), Mike co-founded Back Up, an international charity based in London, which has raised 30 million pounds since its inception, for which he has been paid zero income.

Conversations with Mike inevitably gravitate towards new and future projects— Mike's heartfelt articulation of perpetual motion. But recently he surprised me with uncharacteristic backward motion. Mike's projects are audacious, often fuelled by adrenalin-like excitement, and are only doable because he makes up his mind to do them. Mike is not about to let up on forward motion, but he confided to me that as he gets older he wants to spend more time on Back Up. Though 35 years are in the rear-view mirror, Mike sees a future growing Back Up into an international juggernaut. I agreed that his plan has both excitement and forward motion but felt compelled to warn Mike that if he is not careful he is going to be accused of becoming generous in his late middle years.

You'd think driving around the world and through barriers others never think about—let alone face down and conquer—coupled with that tempering factor called age would cure Mike of lusting for adventurous travel, and yes, predictably, you'd be wrong. As the world tilts from independent travel and real adventure towards comfort, ease, and predictability, Mike has ramped up his travel ambitions. He notes that real adventure is not possible for most people with significant disabilities, and Mike's ambition is to always make possible the impossible, even for those who do not share his ambition. Mike reasons Canadian winters are far too long for people with mobility impairments and escapes in spectacular fashion. After driving around the world, the winter escape is no big deal. From northern latitudes of eastern Canada, Mike drives to southern Mexico, and then, ambition unfulfilled, he reasons that Costa Rica is only a stone's throw away.

And it is here that he finds a way to fulfill his travel ambition. Mike is currently pursuing what he describes as *his most ambitious project ever*, so you've got to pay attention. He is intending to develop "remote resorts"—that is, seven fully accessible, full service, five-star resorts—in four continents over the next 20 years. Though Mike may or may not be successful, his most ambitious project ever has to be taken seriously to have any understanding of the man who refused to let losing everything amount to anything.

When we talk, he might say something about his project's progress or, just as likely, not. If not, it doesn't mean it's not. Asking him about any project underway always results in breathtaking audacity and detail, except when it has been dropped for something bigger. Dropping a project is never a loss, just a detail, a thing of the past in a world where future plans are so much more interesting. Mike emphasizes that he learns far more from his failures than his successes. Makes sense—obtaining glory tends not to be a great teacher, gratifying as it might feel.

Mike is a nice guy, but you don't want to be the barrier that prevents him from doing what he has set out to do. Six federally chartered banks found out that Mike can be as ferocious as a wolverine when he took them to the Canadian Human Rights Commission over a ten-year period, forcing them to collectively redesign their ATM machines. Before he undertook his transformation of the financial world, Mike had to rely on a paid attendant to use a banking machine, thereby surrendering his independence, privacy, and, as it turns out, money. Not being a stickler about money, Mike did not at first notice that his trusted attendant was systematically robbing him. Mike got mad—a not good thing or a really great thing, depending—and decided to act. Though it took some real time—the banks do have power, after all—the banks relented and were required to spend over 900 million dollars to make ATMs accessible. There's a rumour that the banks petitioned to have the next major hurricane named Hurricane Mike. Okay, so I started the rumour, but there are likely more than a few bankers who would have willingly signed the petition.

One day between projects, Mike heard that a couple of us were going to the governor general's reception to see Rick Hansen receive the Order of Canada. Mike decided to come along. If Rick Hansen could make a career and create an empire out of his Man in Motion Tour, at a time when people were far less aware of disability issues, Mike had the drive to put his drive into the passing lane. At the reception Mike approached Rick, who was wearing his Order of Canada medal and was presumably in a generous state of mind. Mike asked Rick to support his Round the World aspirations, and since they had in common raising funds for spinal cord research, it seemed a natural fit. But for whatever reason, Rick was not interested in Mike's plans, was not interested in becoming one of Mike's best pals, was just not interested. Rick could not be convinced to paint Mike's fence and to pay for the privilege. This was competition, not co-operation, and Mike did not appreciate the slight.

For all his big plans, Mike always has another bigger one in the wings just in case things don't work out, and the unavoidable truth is, things usually don't. Mike approaches another, bigger celebrity, with more clout, with whom he instantly becomes best pals. Christopher Reeve had a horseback riding accident in 1995, instantly becoming a high-level (C-1) quadriplegic—as high a level as is possible and still be alive. Rather than mix it up with self-indulgent Hollywood types post-accident, Christopher devoted himself to spinal cord awareness and research. Mike and Christopher became a genuine mutual admiration society, did much together, and would have done much more if Chris had not died a few years later. (For example, Chris was just three weeks away from narrating Mike's Round the World Challenge documentary when he died.) Mike attended Chris's 50th birthday fundraising dinner in Times Square, New York City.

Chris then came to Ottawa for his good friend Mike's Round the World Challenge fundraising gala. At the end of the evening they shared the stage together, displaying the power of friendship and connection in service to a cause greater than themselves, the capacity audience tingling in witness to their authentic, poignant bond. Both men spoke powerfully, convincingly, and if Mike's Round the World Challenge truck had been waiting outside the building, I might have abandoned wife and kids at that moment to tour with Mike, but it was not, and lucky for me. I remember clearly, vividly, time in perpetuity that night, most of all and forever Christopher's heartfelt most quotable mantra: "So many of our dreams at first seem impossible, then they seem improbable, and then, when we summon the will, they soon become inevitable."

After the speeches—less talking heads than Churchillian oratory—a surprise. Christopher Reeve was Superman to millions after starring in a film by the same name in 1978, written by Mario Puzo, with three Superman sequels to follow. Reeve's subsequent actions as a quadriplegic who refused to be defeated only reinforced his "superman" persona. From a 1991 album, a Canadian band called the Crash Test Dummies had a big hit called "Superman's Song." It became strongly associated with the Superman of the four Hollywood films and, most of all, the man known as Christopher Reeve. The song was distinctive because of the bass-baritone vocals of singer-songwriter Brad Roberts. As the Ottawa gala came to a close, with Christopher and Mike holding the stage, Brad Roberts walked out singing "Superman's Song" to the number one and number two supermen on the planet. A fitting close to an evening etched forever in the minds of the more than 800 who had the privilege to attend the super evening.

At the time and often since I've wondered if Chris knew that his inspiring words would never apply to him. For all his good looks, superpowers, fame, and money, he must have known nothing could save him. And yet there he was paying it forward, telling us to embrace the evolution of hope from impossible to improbable to inevitable. He must have known that a breakthrough, the inevitability factor from dream to solving traumatic spinal injury, was many years in the future. Not long after the gala of hope, gracious determination succumbed to the inevitability of his condition. For now, very high-level quadriplegics tend to have compromised longevity. Chris died, age 52, a portrait of tragic courage, followed the following year by the unexpected death of his young wife, Dana Reeve, age 44—a lifelong non-smoker—from lung cancer. Curious footnote about the death of this most glamorous Hollywood power couple: we obsess today about privilege, fame, and money, forgetting that no amount of it can save us from material-world brute forces. If there is nothing beyond the great pale, banishing the nightmare of our dreams is "impossible," the meaning of love and loss, "improbable," seeking solace in nihilistic world distraction, "inevitable." For all the disparity and unfairness of this life, it comes to the same inclusive and equitable place, and that too is inevitable. It just might be that seeking our material-world advantage is not the point of it all.

And this. Being dealt such nasty cards, it does seem a tough place from which to be generous. To fall from his horse, as a rich, handsome Hollywood A-lister, into the vacuum of restriction and loss that became his life would seem to logically engender despair and bitterness. But Christopher Reeve chose, again chose, consciously, intentionally, painfully to be other than logic engenders. With obvious application to his own life, Chris had this to say about his friend Mike Nemesvary: "In a moment, in a heartbeat, your life can change. And yet, you find when it changes that there are reserves of strength, reserves of resourcefulness, reserves of energy that you can call on to go forward … Nobody exemplifies that better than Mike." When all is bad, when despair looms, when faith fades, there is the pervasive "and yet…" forging of the soul for possibility from Christopher Reeve.

Mike's natural bent towards taking life by the horns, his bravado, audacity, and single-mindedness, has cost him. His drive to jump higher on that trampoline when he probably shouldn't have been jumping at all cost him everything he valued in life; it cost him glamour, career options, relationships, mobility, and the ability to simply get out of a chair and walk into whatever the world has to offer at any given moment in time. Mostly, and publicly, Mike talks about overcoming barriers, changing attitudes, planning big projects, completing big projects, and the next big projects, always doing what needs to be done in order not to be outdone. Without necessarily intending to, Mike evokes his inner Superman as the requisite persona to defeating the villains of defeatism.

Even in his most vulnerable moments, Mike stays in control, does not fully relinquish the ability to do anything. Most people can't even vaguely imagine Mike's life; fewer still can imagine getting themselves out of the very real ordeals of his life. In a piece Mike wrote called "Forty Hours in Bed," he dispassionately recounts a mix-up with an attendant, the failure of his electronic security system, and just bad timing, which, taken together, almost killed him. He was unceremoniously dropped off by a friend after a New Year's Eve party, quickly thrown into bed, and forgotten for 40 hours, during which time, time seemed to stop. While Mike contemplated his dismal circumstances, it was not clear if he would be discovered until after his death. Slow as it was, time did painstakingly inch forward, but with growing awareness of dehydration, hunger, distended bowels, increasing muscle spasticity leading to the potential for deadly autonomic dysreflexia, the smell of his own urine and feces, head cold and headache, the inability to raise his own voice, and wavering cognitive functioning. Inexplicably, in the toxic mix was the emerging possibility of being eaten alive by his pet cat, whose behaviour under changed circumstances took on a malevolent nature.

This is a portrait in vulnerability, humiliation, and hopelessness, and yet, it is not how Mike interpreted his situation. Mike, who does not talk about God, "said a little prayer and asked my higher power to see me through this horror. I then promised myself that I would deal with my situation without panicking."

Later, listening to Mike retell the ordeal, matter-of-factly, as is his way, I again felt an unreasonable stirring of claustrophobia and panic. From my risk-free uninvolved perch of listening and taking notes, I also felt a bit embarrassed. *What a wimp*, I thought of me, and *How the hell did he do it*? I thought of Mike. It is one thing to make a courageous choice during the light of day, to an admiring audience; it is quite another to steel oneself, only to oneself, to endure, whatever might come, with toughness and integrity, facing the prospect of dying painfully, shortly, and alone.

Another curious dimension of Mike's stoic courage is that in the 25 years I have known him, he has never asked, whispered, or hinted at the obvious and, at some level, compelling question: *Why me*? Not asking the why me question is perhaps healthy, or even a necessary ingredient to survival, and may be the most admirable aspect of his character. And this is the heart or spirit of the matter, for Mike's story is not really an adventure story so much as it is a profound mystery that begs for understanding. Courage is the wilful expression, but not quite the essence.

In all the years I've known him, Mike has never mentioned belief in a higher power, and I'd never asked. But once I'd read that he offered up a prayer during his 40-hour ordeal, I decided to ask him. We were sitting in his backyard in the spring sun after an unusually tough Ottawa winter, which are always tough, and toughest of all for people with mobility impairments. For Mike the *toughest of all* winter scenario had been ratcheted up further still by a blood clot that had been ignored, that had refused to be ignored, that had almost killed him. He was slowly recovering; slower still was his recovery from many weeks in hospital. And as often happens, Mike had had the ironic and sadly common experience of catching a worse infection in hospital while being treated for a lesser one. For a while it looked like he was going to lose his leg just below the knee. Again, the irony, Mike notes, before adding, "which made me afraid that I'd never walk again."

On this day we sat outside, sun seeking and squinting, talking and shivering, because for all the medicinal benefits of sunlight, it was still bloody cold. We took in the expanse of green, a nice change from our white winter of discontent, surveying past the large property to the golf course beyond. Mike's backyard meets the golf course at the junction of the fourth and fifth hole, that too continuing the irony theme because his catastrophic spinal cord injury was at the junction of his fourth and fifth vertebrae. On this day Mike laughs at this juxtaposition with his weakened laugh, the prospect of death recently having receded, though never out of mind, and he is in an exceedingly rare philosophical mood. He answers in the affirmative the one time I ask, "Sure, it makes sense that God exists," and we leave it at that.

But as to that, I can't leave it at that. It is my pathetic way to excavate the un-answered questions of the ten-year-old boy within. Why is suffering so spectacularly uneven and unfair, and why is our response to it so flat? If there is no purpose in suffering, nihilism wins and life is sad and meaningless. Actually, if meaninglessness rules, even sad is irrelevant since all human emotion amounts to nothing. For many, or perhaps sadly most (sadly applying only to those who have not capitulated to nihil-ism), the question needn't be asked or dwelt upon. It just is. For the minority plagued by the relevance of emotions such as sadness, the question must be asked, even if the answer is slow to lifelong in coming: What is the meaning of suffering?

For many, meaning has to do with personal comfort, self-actualization, and accumulation of stuff. In other words, there is no preoccupation with meaning in suffering; rather, meaning is extracted from the avoidance of suffering. Suffering then being antithetical to meaning, and since we can never hold comfort together forever, we of necessity arrive at nihilism. Our individual pursuits are avoidance, and life is denial.

Which seems to work for most people, though pulling off collective denial is a daunting task. Even if we temporarily ignore that the grim reaper is on his way, there are seven billion of us making our way through this life, with over 14 times that number having preceded us. Comfort in our own singularity is cold comfort and is likely why denial is enmeshed in over-arching collective human ennui. We cannot unknow what we know, and it is knowing and not comfort that pervades our dreams.

I could ruminate and muse for a thousand years on how Mike can shrug his shoulders (below which he has no feeling) and kid about having diminished mobility if he lost his leg. Sure, I am amazed and humbled by Mike's strength—like Peter's, Gord's, and so many others'—his ability to reframe perpetual suffering into casual and commonplace. And as we do in those philosophical moments, Mike and I talk about the reality of struggle as a quadriplegic, wherein no amount of habit and adaptation changes the immediacy and extremity of restriction. But endurance alone cannot be meaning. Rather, endurance alone, admirable as it is, argues for meaninglessness.

I admire and marvel at Mike's courage without much understanding, though I believe it must mean something, must mean much. For most of us, our lived experience among humanoid fragments of consciousness is separateness. But there is more. In rare moments when we do not take it for granted, consciousness is also, and ultimately, a portal to a shared version of a dimly suspected life, the potential for self-evident truth that can only be explained as admission of existence of the soul.

Which, if it exists, does change things. That is, accessing rare moments in search for self-evident truths might begin to yield something of meaning. If suffering is universal and unrelenting, it must exist for a reason, must be a necessary fact of life. If the self-evidence of the soul exists as a communion rather than a separation of humanity, then the uneven prevalence of suffering lends itself to the notion of shared necessity, and therefore those who suffer most contribute most to the well of collective human suffering. Maybe absorption of suffering, the act of sacrifice from personal experience—say Mike's 40 hours, Jesus's 40 days and 40 nights—alleviates individual suffering for others.

Maybe Mike's 18 trips to the World Cup circuit skiing podium is not the basis of his heroism. (Mike may read this and be appalled at how little detail and drama I have given to his great adventures. But that is his story, which he is writing, and not mine.) What interests me about Mike's story is beyond athleticism, and to my mind the accessing of higher self is higher than stepping up to the podium to accept the medal, the one that still pervades his dreams, that he never got to compete for in the 1992 Olympics. I know that the narrative dog bites man is easier to believe than man bites dog, but the latter really is more compelling. Mike has always done the hard thing, gone against the grain, been the man who bites the dog. Still, with apologies to my friend, we have to disagree. Sorry, Mike, but your life is more than besting speed records, beating the banks, or building world-class accessible resorts, even though you may argue the case once your book comes out.

Mike used to soar from earth's shackles into liberating sky from atop the highest mountains. Chris used to soar through air, cape flapping in the wind, as he flew to where he was destined to foil the next dastardly criminal. Both doing what they were meant to do, in full control, whom we admired most, and whom we most wanted to be. But we, the adoring fans, moved on because we didn't want them to become like us—vulnerable, flawed, without magic. Common tragic figures.

Still, some few have super vision, can see beyond material-world restriction, to what lies ahead, to whomever is placed along their path. Mike and Chris played heroic roles, their movies ended, and they became supermen in the movie adaptation called life. They soar from the heights of their higher selves still.

Chapter Ten

DO-MANCE OF THE CENTURY

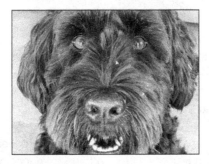

"All his life he tried to be a good person. Many times, however, he failed. For after all, he was only human. He wasn't a dog."
Charles M. Schulz, cartoonist, creator of Snoopy (1922–2000)

We humans have a strange relationship with animals. We use them and eat them, we befriend them and revere them, and we see no contradiction in this. They submissively allow us to have our way with them, rarely eat us, and seem to love us even as we do the most unlovable things for which humans are renowned. I am a serial dog guy, a confession made earlier in *Lament for Spilt Porter*. I wrote about Sonny, our Portuguese water dog, in that book, and he being Cara's dog, he remains a grumpy but robust Cara-canine of 16 years. He never did learn how to like water and still cannot speak Portuguese. Even his claim to being a dog is open to dispute based on his curmudgeonly old man behaviour, but that is another story.

We also have a six-year-old Portuguese, Zigo, named after my childhood imaginary friend, and he has always been, decidedly, *my* dog. Bitcoin bribes didn't work, so I won Zigo over by taking him on daily runs, beginning at four months old and continuing until today. And he's become a bit of a neighbourhood celebrity since he runs by my side off leash through city streets in a way most dogs can never do. (On a sample of one, Sonny would have preferred to take tango lessons with the neighbour cat than run with me, let alone manage to do so off leash.)

Running with Zigo is a nice change from several decades of competitive road racing. All these years it has never been clear to me if my former brutal training regime was about exercising muscles or exorcising my demons. In recent years, I've realized there are more challenging exercises than exhausting limbs and lungs. Whether or not with pal Zigo, we are called upon to exercise the potential of consciousness, including our many inarticulate ruminations, to figure out if this life has any meaning. And though marathons, yoga studios, and kale consumption promise incalculable benefits, modernity is noteworthy for its palpable resistance to spiritual exercise. It seems our sense of possibility and willingness to live with uncertainty are contracting.

If you are unable to reconcile yourself to spiritual doubt for physical world certainty, try this: go on a walk or wheel and consider the world—that is, without your smartphone. Think about the big questions and your own lonely existence. Breathe as you walk or roll and feel your muscles in motion reminding you that *This is it, baby, here and now*. Look around, take it all in, the sights, sounds, and smells. Keep moving, and first think of artistry and mystery, details in every direction, then that everything and every detail comes to nothing. Think about the concept of love as one and indivisible in perpetuity, and then as applied to the singular phenomenology of who you love. Think cells temporarily alive, followed by death and oblivion. Repeat.

Now try to imagine your own non-existence—not death; that is relatively easy—I mean imagine never having existed non-existence, which is the reality of the atheistic world. If you can't conceive of your own non-existence (the curse and blessing of consciousness is that we cannot), then the atheist belief that having died would be the same as never having lived is a lie. So, why do you believe in what is untrue even as you feel existence pumping through your veins with each purposeful stride or wheel up the incline scattering autumn leaves with sunlight streaming through a thousand narrow corridors delighting movement with infinitesimal change and possibility? And life.

Continue on with just the possibility of God in mind—stop resisting; this is only an exercise while you exercise, after all. Suspend deciding whether or not you believe in God—I'm fairly certain that God's existence or non-existence isn't dependent upon what any of us decides—and allow in the tiny perfect thought that maybe, just maybe, life does not end with death. Allow in a bit of well-earned relief, just for a moment. Who doesn't crave relief from certain oblivion? Don't worry what continued life might be—much of what is wrong with materialism is the inability to accept uncertainty as the reality of life. And don't sweat not knowing our purpose— maybe purpose is approaching life with an open heart and open mind, being open to receiving glimpses of spiritual revelation. Whatever is to be revealed in death, it will probably knock us over with its utter simplicity. Like remembering someone's long forgotten name in the middle of the night or the punchline to a joke you couldn't quite recall that afternoon. You think, *Of course, that's it*!

Openness—without expectation of knowing—may fit purpose by allowing us to see and come to understand the reality of the miracle beneath the mundane.

If everything hangs on God and if consciousness is our vehicle for awareness, supplemented by an attitude of openness, miracles are wherever we look. Dawkins's "gaps" may be not-solvable problems—that is, once science gets to them. Rather, they may not be gaps at all but proof of God's existence, and our failure to see gaps as such may be wilful blindness. Openness—cultivating wonder and experiencing awe—may be what this brief physical life has to offer, and for those not married to the human conceit of knowing all, it is enough. Gaps are God, and purpose is knowing this.

When *Lament for Spilt Porter* was launched, our local television station did a profile, and being a visible medium, they wanted a shot of me running. When they heard that in recent years I do my daily running with pal Zigo, they thought it might be cute. I warned them that Zigo's enthusiasm for our running communion has not flagged in the five years and eight months since we started, and his enthusiasm might be a tad distracting. Roll camera, and there he was, unprompted, not running so much as jumping up on two legs with every stride, less man's best friend than Tigger bouncing on his tail through the Hundred Acre Woods. It would have been impossible to make him stop, even though it was a noontime fake shot and Zigo had had his actual run at 6:30 a.m., that, and every, morning.

The television guys thought it was beyond cute and a keeper. Same for a still shot, sitting on a bench in the park behind my house (which I had never actually done before), whereupon Zigo immediately went up on two legs and laid his front paws on my arm, for a spectacular visual still, which is no more than he always does. Same for sitting, watching TV, or any time I am still; Zigo has to sit beside me with his paws on my arm or leg, anything as long as contact is made and maintained. When I'm driving my truck, he comes forward from the backseat into the middle section where I am changing gears, and he rests his paws on my right forearm, and no amount of disruption—which when you are driving a manual transmission vehicle happens every few seconds—can convince him that he should not try, yet again, to make and maintain contact. And I think—he's a bit weird, kind of obsessive, and surely the greatest dog who has ever lived.

As for my weird and obsessive attachment to him, I have to admit that when I travel and wake up a bit disoriented in a strange room, my first impulse is to wonder where Zigo is, since he always sleeps beside me at home. Well, Cara sleeps beside me at home too, but I am a wee bit ashamed that her absence only springs to mind a millisecond after Zigo's—not much time, but still second place. Then again, she probably wakes up when I'm away and thinks, *Oh good, as long as Zigo is here*.

While I am unapologetically biased in favour of Zigo in particular, dogs in general, and most any pet great and small, it must be said that Zigo, dogs, and pets are not therapists. I am not attempting to assign them to a lesser role, but like many, I have become perplexed. For all my years as director of the Paul Menton Centre we had students with service dogs that provided essential services (hence the designation) for students with disabilities. These dogs were carefully selected for calm temperament—with most puppies not making the cut—and trained to a rigorous standard over a period of many months. They are working animals, capable of doing specific tasks, and whose behaviour is impeccable to the point of becoming invisible in a crowd of people.

Guide dogs are the exemplar, allowing people who are completely blind to find destinations and avoid barriers, without death or injury ensuing. Some service dogs can be trained to perform tasks for other disabilities, including physical and psychiatric conditions. Mike Nemesvary's dog Jigger helps retrieve items that he cannot reach or pick up because of his limited hand dexterity. Jigger is calm and composed in all situations, including when Mike ran over his tail with his 200-pound wheelchair. Ouch. Jigger now has a stump, which limits his ability to wag his tail, but being a well-trained service dog, he never did get much chance for such frivolity, so no great loss. In the lawsuit against Mike, Jigger described his physical loss as causing a "wag-ability," but in the end he dropped the case out of love for his sheepish owner. Mike still feels bad; Jigger, apparently not so much. As far as we know, dogs are not capable of resentment. Just part of the service, ma'am.

It is no exaggeration to claim our animal relationships of such importance that they provide an answer to the existential question regarding what it is to be human. Still, across North America a strange thing has happened. Changes have been made to legislation to forgo the standard of service dogs and expand rights to the unregulated therapy and emotional support animal categories, and yes, that would be animals in the plural writ large, so cats and rats and elephants have the potential to be included in our endless quest to be inclusive.

What the animal is trained to do, is capable of doing, and how the animal behaves in relation to the entire world into which he or she has been included has been subverted to a generalized ideology of inclusion. And this inclusion exists because of our greater need to include all people who claim to have a condition that necessitates having the comforting inclusion of their animal of choice. This well-intended and poorly thought out expansion of human rights activism has yielded interesting results.

Here are some media highlights. In 2014, a woman carried her emotional support (ES) pig in her carry-on bag on a United Airways flight from Connecticut to Washington. The woman was able to get her pig through the airline ticket counter and security because she had followed the proper emotional support animal protocol. It was universally acknowledged that the pig stank to high heaven, though olfactory consideration of all other passengers was never going to result in its expulsion. That only happened when the pig defecated on the floor, as pigs tend to do, and often, hence the pejorative association with the name of the animal.

In 2016, a passenger was allowed to take her ES turkey on a Delta flight. In the same year, Daniel, an ES duck, became something of a celebrity on a flight after being photographed wearing stylish red shoes and a Captain America diaper. A university student flushed her ES hamster down the toilet after Spirit Airlines refused to accommodate Pebbles, as the student chose the spring break flight over her beloved animal. There was some controversy as to whose idea it was to permanently waterboard poor young Pebbles, but Spirit Airlines took the situation seriously enough to issue a formal statement, denying that the woman "was instructed to flush the animal down the toilet." Continuing along, a doctor from York wrote a support letter approving Wally the alligator for travel as an alternative to medication.

Fast forward a bit. In May 2019, poor Kokito, an ES French bulldog, died in an overhead bin on a United Airlines Flight. Poor Kokito was relegated to the overhead bin because there has been some recent concern that the emotional support movement might have become a tad bit excessive. Same for a woman on a British Airways flight who caused a commotion when she tried to smuggle her cat onboard in October 2018. As well, a New York performance artist posted a photo of her peacock at the airport along with this: "Spent 6 hours trying to get a flight to LA (after following all required protocol). Tomorrow my human friends are going to drive me cross country. Keep an eye out for us. #bestroadtripbuddy #dexterthepeacock." In October 2018, a woman was told to either leave or face arrest on a Frontier Airlines flight after the airline refused to accommodate her squirrel, Daisy. The woman was distraught: "You will not take my baby from me."

After which Frontier changed its policy, stipulating that an emotional support animal must be either a dog or a cat. American Airlines has a list of disqualified animals, including amphibians, snakes, hedgehogs, non-household birds, and animals with tusks, horns, or hooves (there was that incident with a kangaroo in Beaver Dam, Wisconsin)—except for miniature horses, which are allowed according to the Americans with Disabilities Act.

However, the proliferation of emotional support animals into every societal nook and cranny extends far beyond air travel, as evidenced by a recent *New York Times* headline: "People are Taking Emotional Support Animals Everywhere." The article profiles a contentious case involving a 26-year-old Starbucks barista and his quest to keep his snow-white duck, Primadonna, from being evicted from his apartment in a Tampa, Florida, suburb. Primadonna's owner has medical notes, in the plural, indicating his need for an emotional support animal, but the landlord insisted that the bird go, which resulted in a legal battle—this being just one of more than 1,000 throughout the U.S. in 2019.

Of course, differentiating between the family pet that no one thinks much about and the idealized version of an animal with curative powers requires a process. A doctor's note may be required, or perhaps a prescription, such as for Wally the alligator by the good doctor from York. With doctors being in high demand, and with busy doctors increasingly acting as patient advocates, and with emotional support animals being a thing, getting a doctor's note is no big deal. People sometimes produce letters after one phone call or quick visit to a never-seen-before doctor at a walk-in clinic.

Until recently, the American PetSmart website noted, "As long as your mental health professional signs off on them, virtually any animal can be an ESA. Technically, sugar gliders and miniature horses could become ESAs." (Don't worry, you're not alone—I had to look up what a sugar glider was; it's a nocturnal gliding possum that when gliding looks a like a bat. Ouch, the sugar glider cannot be a popular post-COVID choice.)

Today, the PetSmart website defers and links to the National Service Animal Registry for information about service and emotional support animals. As recently as 2011, NSAR had a paltry 2,400 emotional support animals in its registry, and today that number is over 200,000, and growing. NSAR focuses on the proliferation of the emotional support designation, which is quite different from the traditional service animal. While the service animal's training standard remains high, the emotional support animal does not require any training at all. Coupled with this revelation is the fact that everyone seems to qualify for an ESA. "An individual is qualified as determined by a mental health professional who has determined that the patient's mental health will be benefited through the companionship of an emotional support animal." For clarity, take out the word *patient* and replace with *human*. The untrained animal with the untrained human is nice, but does it need a formal process?

At which point I have to be clear—I am *not* disparaging the communion between animal and human. In fact, and emphatically, I am for *more* of said communion, but with the added ingredient of common sense. And even as I point out some of the silly activist incidents, I am not against emotional support or therapy designations to the extent that they serve a companionable purpose and help us lowly humans make it through the day. Still, I question the way humans ubercomplicate our animal relationships, since much of their value is as exemplars of simple.

Sandra Oh, as Dr. Christina Yang in *Grey's Anatomy*, repeatedly tells Dr. Meredith Grey, "You're my person." Zigo is my person. But he is not my therapist. The Oxford definition of therapy is "treatment intended to relieve or heal a disorder"; a therapist is "a person skilled in a particular kind of therapy"; and a therapeutic alliance is "the relationship between a psychologist or psychotherapist and a patient, regarded as important for the outcome of psychological therapy." Hum, seems a psycho-babble-centric way to describe the relationship between man and mutt. So why are canines, cats, and ferrets now therapists? Because to get beyond the specialness gate of access to all things, there is a requirement that we identify the human's condition and declare the animal capable of the cure.

Same for the emotional support designation—that is, we pathologize with the connotation that humans will fall apart if not for the emotional support of their wise and venerable animals. Seems like a lot of responsibility for the unknowing, uninterested, and possibly unwilling animal. Sure, Zigo and I have a mutual emotional support thing going on, along with our mutual admiration society. But why do I have to declare having a condition in order to pull it off? Why can't I just declare that he is my person, and I, his, and leave it at that? All successful relationships have an element of mutual emotional support, and it is the two-way element of the support that is key to its success and longevity.

When the emotional support relationship is pathologized, it requires a "special" designation for those who qualify over those who don't, with the potential for absurdities such as a woman bringing a pig onto a plane, in full olfactory assault to all passengers, and no one dares say a word. Also, in order to justify having a pig on a plane, the woman has to declare that being separated from her beloved would result in psychological damage. Between humans, even those who are married, we discourage codependency. With our special animals, codependency is deemed necessary, virtuous even, with a doctor's note to prove it.

Still. Animals fulfill a deep human need that we don't seem to be able to achieve within our own species, and that is weird. On a crowded planet, whether due to or despite social media, people increasingly find it difficult to find meaningful humanoid companions, and yet we enjoy authentic friendship with our resident animal. Lifelong friends are rare, and finding a life/romantic partner is the central fodder for books and movies; such is our obsession with the one and only. We can talk to our pets in a rarified manner, and we can confess things that we would have trouble admitting to ourselves. The fact that their superior listening skills don't necessarily result in comprehension of anything we have said is a minor detail. They know us and don't let a little thing like understanding words deter from that essential fact. (Of course, their combination of listening and incomprehension may make them exemplars of Van Morrison's Shavian saying from which the title *Inarticulate Speech of the Heart* is taken: communicating with as little articulation as possible while at the same time being emotionally articulate.)

If the mixing of human and hamster can help to heal psychological wounds, then it stands to reason that the same relationship also has the potential to provide a powerful antidote to life's vicissitudes. Our pets (sorry for the lowly designation) have the potential to help all of us all the time, and not just some of us when/if we have a condition. Helping to prevent mental illness seems just as important as helping to manage good mental health. Why diagnosis, why stigmatize, why not just admit that the lowly pet can best the best therapist and let in the love? Which results in my long-winded bottom-line question, as follows: Why is Zigo confined to the doghouse because he can't produce a doctor's note about my condition rather than laying his head on my lap as I work in the office, this day, every day, all day long?

Zigo and his many contemporaries are exemplars of relationship, whether or not we give them therapy or emotional designations. The infinite number of complex ways to tank relationships that humans are capable of are absent from animal existence. They are unacknowledged, unappreciated exemplars of simple. Clearly, they are responsible for much that is good about humans, and what is good about humans exists to the extent that we transcend our physical world exteriors and allow in a glimpse of our higher selves. If the pet designation seems too plain, why not call our relationship exemplars "spiritual support animals"?

The wonky elevation of pet to the specialness of therapist may be one of the many material-world outcomes that inevitably creeps into the spiritual space we moderns have vacated. As Victor Frankl observed decades ago, "Depression, aggression, and addiction are not understandable unless we recognize the existential vacuum underlying them." "Spiritual support animal," though less credentialed, seems so much more dignified somehow.

Most kids growing up understood the concept of a guardian angel, and it was comforting to think that there was a spiritual presence that personally knew us, loved us, and looked out for us. That presence helped assuage the pull towards isolation and possible despair that is endemic to the human condition. As adults we throw off childish things, including and perhaps especially the silly concept of a protective guardian angel. But the specialness of relationship with our animals cannot accurately be described as codependent, emotionally supportive, or therapeutic. Animals have in them inherent goodness, and as for humans, well, let's just say we are a work in progress. Our little spiritual support pals are closer to being our guardian angels than therapy-anything because they give us the grace and courage to face this life in which we inexplicably find ourselves. Oh yeah, and because they need their twice daily constitutional, they help us greet whomever God places on our path with wagging tail and open heart.

Postscript: Though it was long anticipated, we suddenly had to put Sonny down. It was crushing. Cara suffered too but for whatever reason was more resolute, knowing it was time. I could not fully accept, irrational as it might be, that we took our trusting dog to his unknowing death, even if it was on the strong advice of the vet. Decision made—out of love but feeling the opposite—Sonny was prepared and sedated by nice, caring staff. But I felt panic, dread even, because while having to wait for over three hours for the vet assessment, Sonny had not been fed. I know how silly this seems, and yet it haunts me. For the past two years he had wasted terribly even as we fed him increasingly more, and for all his maladies, the skinny lad never lost his appetite.

Stroking Sonny, Cara and I each offered him a biscuit, and, God love him, he managed to lift a weary head and enthusiastically gobble them down. I had grabbed three biscuits from the counter and had two more waiting, but before he could eat another, he was gone. I stood like a dolt, uncertain, looking at my hand, wondering what I was going to do with the remaining biscuits.

I left feeling I'd failed Sonny because he had not been properly fed as had been our twice daily ritual for 16 years. When we got home I immediately went to feed Zigo, picked up two bowls to fill with kibble, and then, heavy with dog bowl redundancy, I lost it.

I could say grief is not rational, but it would be more honest to argue for its logic. You see, for all my pathetic attempts at caring, I needed him. I needed to look after him; I needed to fill his bowl as he filled my soul. He was along my path, and the extraordinary thing is, his death reminds me that despair does not emanate from dealing with a crowded path, but rather it is the void we experience when we are alone upon it. Though Sonny was ostensibly Cara's dog, and we always jokingly competed for his attention, we know relationships are sacred regardless of pathetic owner rivalry. Even more than I miss him who loved Cara most, I miss the sacred us that looked after each other along our intersecting paths.

Chapter Eleven

A TWO-HEADED MONSTER CALLED LOVE

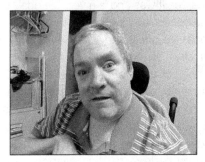

"I hold it true, whatever befall:
I feel it, when I sorrow most;
'tis better to have loved and lost
Than never to have loved at all."
Alfred Lord Tennyson (1809–1892)

Maybe. Of course, Lord Tennyson was a romantic poet and, well, believed in things romantic. We moderns are less enamoured with the romantic poets' version of romance—deep, transporting feelings of agony and ecstasy, characterized by anticipation and denial, all of which is antithetical to the realizing of wants and desires. We don't lose ourselves in the ideal, the other; we find ourselves either satisfied or not satisfied, and if not fully satisfied, we seek romance elsewhere. Still, some few romantics remain.

Doug could perhaps be forgiven for this one spectacularly grievous and unmodern flaw. It caused him to abandon the faculty of reason, a lifelong habit of being reasonable, of seeking shelter within predicable limitations, what could be depend upon, what easily could be known. It was what his mother had him trained to do, and he had always done what his mother told him to do.

And he'd mastered logical and predictable for all his years, right up until he made his one colossal, illogical mistake. Yes, Doug could be forgiven and was by most who read about his mistake years later. But in every waking hour and every solitary moment of sleep during his many nights of self-recrimination, he cried, "How could I be so stupid!"

Maybe beneath the most patent realist beats the inarticulate heart of a romantic, even if the world thinks otherwise. Doug and I remember his first day on campus—we agreed in recent conversation at his apartment one bitterly cold supposedly spring day—about 30 years earlier. That meeting was filled with fear and trepidation, all heightened by the fact that for students with high-level physical disabilities coming from the certainty of their moms' care and cooking into our distant city campus service there exists a minefield of uncertainty. And given that our attendant program was the only game in this or any town, for students like Doug it was possibly their only shot at creating a career. It was and is a very big deal.

On that first day, and continuing for all the years of Doug's education, his mother was a powerful presence. No one or any one service was ever going to replace her—this is a tough transition for parents too—but she was going to make damn sure that we followed her instructions regarding her son. Fair enough. For some situations apron strings are not cut so much as frayed over time until severed.

Over time and with much give and take, she became satisfied that our service was acceptable, which was a huge concession on her part. And with parental crisis averted, Doug settled into a routine that endured: woken by an attendant at 7 a.m.; morning regime performed, taking approximately 90 minutes, before transfer into electric chair; breakfast in residence cafeteria; travel through university subterranean concrete tunnels—our university's five kilometres a distinguishing feature and defence against winter—to any and all academic buildings to attend class; attending all classes sitting alone in a designated disabled space; attempting to make conversation with familiar faces; trying to show interest to the teaching professor; travelling back through concrete tunnel to attendant program for assistance with washroom before travelling upstairs to residence cafeteria for quick lunch and then back to academic buildings for afternoon class, with repeat attempt to show professor interest and same for other students so they can see he is approachable and not to be avoided; and then back through kilometres of stark concrete, barely making it in time for washroom assistance before going upstairs for dinner (assistance from program attendants for all three meals); same predictable mealtime company with other attendant program residents, with some conversation, a few jokes, but not much lingering even as looking around the big cafeteria to the other world, not so much shut out of as impossible to imagine, and yet there it is—casual people, movement, normalcy, spontaneity, happiness, effortlessly floating by without a deliberate thought about anything except for their shared amusement and preservation of unflawed inaccessible beauty for all to see in the elusive, unconscious moment.

And then to work. Readings, assignments, looming term papers, coming quizzes, all taking more time—Doug's blood, sweat, and tears—but no compromise in quality to achieve the work, the courses, the degree, the holy grail. At 10 p.m. the attendant hour ritual begins, with 11 p.m. time enough for bed, a long day, another long one next day, and the day after, the routine constant as the sun and moon rising and falling with flawless predictability, as is his life—mother rest assured. For all the adherence to routine, Doug wants it known that he could not have graduated or had a career without the attendant services program in residence. In his last two years of an intense degree, he routinely had to break routine, working long into the evening in order to succeed. He says that the attendants always allowed him the flexibility he needed, for which he will be eternally grateful. Doug's sincerity is touching, though it exposes him as thoroughly unmodern for his inability to take things for granted.

Four years pass, and in predictable fashion Doug graduates top of his class with a marketable business degree and manages to get a good government job. The job is not easy, but it is work in his field; it is secure and within his comfort zone. He has an accessible apartment with attendant service. He is secure and independent. He is, in short, a success story.

He has friends, too, and is himself a good and loyal friend. No romantic relationships and no expectation that he be in one, certainly not from anyone else. Still, deep down in that inarticulate place, he yearns for a princess, just like everybody else. Always just below the surface, never boiling over, muted disappointment, less expectation than low-grade fever called loneliness, as present and predictable as the attendant who gets him up each morning to go to work. Which raises the question, If all you know is loneliness, is it loneliness or is it something else?

To which Doug articulates about all things sports, mostly on television in his apartment, and with friends, sports spectating being something that spans the divide between guys living precariously through their heroes. Doug reminisces that he originally intended to become a sports journalist, but his mother talked him into pursuing a career that was less risky.

Another 15 years passes, as time predictably does, and we are predictably surprised.

There is nothing wrong. Still, the gnawing to exist, to exit predictable and to really live, not precariously but fully and articulately, does not go away. The need to feel is not assuaged by unfeeling. Passion burned through numbness and loneliness, and in this he was not predictable.

Doug's curse or blessing in this life is that he had to live authentic experiences. But what could he do?

Doug is, to this day, deeply ashamed by what he did. After a lifetime of trying other ways, it is hard to fault him, though he is unaffected by the general moratorium on blame and shame. His take is that he did it, and blame and shame is what he deserves. He hired an escort, and for about a year she provided him with a regular, predictable sexual outlet. It was a satisfactory working relationship, if only it had remained a working relationship. In retrospect, perhaps Doug should reconsider his shame in light of a John O'Donohue saying: "It is human longing that makes us holy."

Two things happened in near proximity that changed Doug's world. Doug's lifetime constant, his mother, became ill. His rock of Gibraltar, a force impossible to replicate, the solution to a lifetime of problems, became *the* problem once they received news that she had cancer. All parents, especially parents of adult children with disabilities, worry about what happens to their children after they are gone. Doug has a sister, and his mom reasoned that between her two children with uneven needs, an uneven distribution of resources would be required, would be fair. Without consulting either of her children, Doug's mother bequeathed Doug sole ownership of the family home. Her daughter would understand, and besides, she had a husband to look after her, whereas Doug was alone.

But Doug's sister did not understand. The ownership of the family home was only revealed after their mother died. Doug's sister was angry and felt betrayed. No worries, Doug responded, he agreed with his sister and would find a way to make things right. Doug's immediate instinct was to protect his relationship with his sister, even if that meant going against the spirit of his mother's will. It was, he reasoned, the right thing to do.

Problem solved, crisis averted. At which precise moment the other thing happened. Well, it less happened than was enacted with precision in order to capitalize on the first thing that had happened. Doug's escort, Dee, knew he had been developing feelings for her. In fact, she had encouraged Doug's feelings, and coyly, cleverly, demurely had let it be known that she too was developing feelings. As well, Doug felt increasingly guilty about paying her, and especially that other men paid her for her services. It wasn't that he minded the expenditure. Rather, he felt that he was acting dishonourably by mixing money and feelings, and he wanted to do the right thing, whatever that was. They both seemed to have come to the end of the escort arrangement. For him, it was the precursor to becoming spectacularly vulnerable; for her and her accomplice, it was the perfect moment to enact their scam.

They were practised fraudsters, and every moment leading to *the* moment was a premeditated attempt to strip Doug of all his worldly possessions. Doug had unique qualities that made him just too good a victim to pass up on: he was naive, trusting, decent, had just fallen in love, and with the death of his mother was both emotionally raw and about to be flush with cash.

Though seemingly unrelated, the prospect of death and the immediacy of sex are often found metaphorically under the sheets together. We crave contact as we lose it. The cessation of material world embodiment compels us towards physical touch while it is possible. The thought of white light effervescence tends not to have the same attraction as physical expression for those who grieve.

Turns out that as Doug's feelings congealed into love, Dee's did too, in harmony, in equal degree, the completion of other, soulmates coming to fruition. It wasn't just business and sex; it was as he had dreamed, love and love-making. It was heaven on earth.

It was hell. Doug had no idea what he was up against. Now that they had an understanding, declarations were fast and furious. Doug had waited a lifetime for his life to begin. Having pledged to spend their lives together, they moved decisively to create one. Being in love, filled with the glow of possibilities, why not create an ideal life? Why be predictable?

They'd had enough of predictable. Predictable work, predictable guys demanding predictable services, and predictable reaction from anyone who knew them if they were to tell them, so they held off talking to people who would not understand their love, who might pierce the bubble of the ideal. She was going to quit demeaning herself as an escort, and he was going to surprise people. They needed a new life, and a new life required a new setting and a new status. They would get married and move away from Ottawa and its cold predictability.

And once engaged (she to be married; he, hook, line, and sinker) she had a detailed plan. Doug was all ears and open wallet. The plan came in three stages. Stage One: They could have it all. She just happened to have a connection in the Dominican Republic, where she just happened to have discovered a fire sale of a small hotel that could double as blissful home and viable business. The coincidences got better. The contact that had the line on the real estate deal of the century was also family. In fact, she had a number of family members who would become his family too, just in case he or anyone should mistake their union as desperate escape rather than pull towards community. They, that is, Doug would never be lonely again. Doug, who had procured a life of boring predictability, was inadvertently on the precipice of unpredictable extraordinaire and had discovered that rarest state of being: happiness. The predator knew her prey well.

Being in a generous state of mind, Doug writes a very substantial check to buy the hotel, because deals like that don't wait around long, and happiness is not for the faint of heart. The deal is that good, just ask her family once they meet. He wants to meet her family, for connection, to make more real the unreality of his happiness, and in his haste to make that happen, Doug gives away everything he owns.

Stage Two: Designed to insert the hook deeper. Which is odd considering the guy has handed over all his money, is all in, cannot go back, does not want to go back. Still, the narrative of the Dominican Republic dream home, the one Doug has paid for, is desperate to get to but will never see, requires additional lies to keep alive. The completion of the scam depends on Doug being able to taste and smell his fictitious home. Dee suggests that they take a trip to the Dominican Republic at Christmas so that Doug can meet her family and see their home — this being the equivalent of using a puppy to lure a child into a waiting van, with even the puppy being a lie. Doug is not only ecstatic; he is determined to win her family over, to make them understand that he is good for Dee, to convince them to become his family too.

And then the absolute completion of happiness, beyond anything he ever hoped for in his wildest, loneliest, private dreams — the one thing that negates all previous loneliness, that nullifies all the men who have ever used Dee, his wife to be, the purist woman who ever lived. And if any hesitation existed before, Dee's news was a direct appeal to Doug's deep decency, responsibility, and most of all, his need to love and be loved, the wellspring of meaning in his life: she is pregnant. Love is blind—that is, it never seemed to occur to Doug that given Dee's history as an escort, the child might not be his.

The days until Christmas count down slowly. Doug wants to tell people everything, but they have agreed not yet. Just a little longer to make sure everything is in place. Twenty sleeps left, fourteen, twelve, nine, seven …

Stage Three: Getting to utopia can be stressful; not for Doug, for he is electric with happiness and hope. But for Dee things are different. After all, it is her vision, her contacts, her family; it was she who found the great real estate deal and proceeded to take care of all the many complex details so that they might have some happiness. But all that sacrifice and effort at creating happiness has cost her. And just to prove that the stress of sacrifice is real, Dee announces—to Doug's bewilderment and disappointment—that she has miscarried their fictitious baby. Poor Doug—he suffers, the more so because at each stage of this fictitious narrative unfolding with the length and complexity of a Tolstoy novel, he could have told people, anyone he trusted, who would most certainly have seen the obvious and told him the truth. Perhaps at some level, in the blissful vortex of deep faux-love, he did not want to know anything that could quell the glow, even, or especially, the truth. Sure, the truth will set you free, free to be lonely, free to be completely devoid of passion, free to exist without hope, free to be predictable. Perhaps for that brief euphoric swirl Doug wanted the truth less than he wanted to live the life of a blissful lie. Apart from Doug, who could blame him?

The newest lie was born of predictable intent. The grifters wanted more. Normally crooks, having extracted all of their victim's money, might conclude that you can't draw blood from a stone and move on. Not quite yet, Dee and Danovan (former husband and present partner in crime) thought; the stone might still yield more if bled properly. Which speaks to the nature of lying and the liar. Scott Peck wrote about the prevalence of evil framed within the banality of the innocuous lie in *People of the Lie*. Winston Churchill famously quipped, "A lie gets halfway around the world before the truth has a chance to get its pants on."

The truth is, the lie mostly wins. In response to Dee's stress and the death of their baby, Doug pleads, "What can I do?" Otherwise put, Doug's How can I serve? How can I be useful? How can I prove my love? pleading sets the stage for his final humiliation.

Dee is coy at first, replying that there is nothing Doug can do. Yet, upon reflection there may be one small thing that would distract her from this tragedy (never mind that the one small thing she is about to ask for is more of what was supposed to have stressed her out to begin with). By serendipitous circumstance, there just happens to be an even better, far less expensive property that has come up for sale in the Dominican Republic. And if she'd seen it before they bought their hotel, she would have chosen this bed and breakfast. Bed and breakfasts are always profitable and easy to sell if you need to. It really doesn't matter that Doug doesn't have the money, not even to Doug. He has offered to extract his own blood from a stone of her choosing and is always good for his word. And the goodness of Doug's word is exactly how the badness of the lie wins. Her argument is for purchasing the real estate opportunity of a lifetime, and his intent is to prove his love for now and all time. Predictably, he finds a way to borrow the money for the second fictitious property. Doug hands over what he doesn't have with a smile, and unbeknownst to him, it is accepted with a figurative smirk.

Doug had wanted to tell his sister about his good fortune, and to do so with an unpredictable sense of flair, for which he was not known. Though by now short of cash, he has paid for his sister and husband to travel to the Dominican Republic with him on December 27th as their special extravagant Christmas present. On Christmas morning with childlike excitement in anticipation of his journey with just two sleeps to go, Doug received an email from Danovan, who pretends to be one of Dee's Dominican Republic family members—though he did so from the safe haven of Jamaica where he had been for the entire scam. Danovan wrote that he is very sorry to inform Doug that Dee has been killed in a car accident.

Doug's first thought is *I can't be this unlucky*, which was both literally true and ironically untrue. Despite his delusional frame of mind, a modicum of truth and sanity flashed before his eyes. Still, revelation is painful. Doug talks poignantly and candidly (the only way he knows how) about how he has barely been able to cope in the 15 or years since that revelation. Almost as difficult as the email he received was having to try to explain to his sister later the same day why they were not going to the Dominican Republic for a holiday—with the full horror of what he had done following in the wake of the first disappointment. Cancelled trip leads to revelations of secrets kept and counsel not sought, fake death, elaborate scam, money lost, inability to rectify Mom's will, sister's rage, estrangement, and years of loneliness and guilt. Doug prays that one day his sister will forgive him. She is all the family he has left.

Just before I read about Doug's ordeal, I had my own revelation or awakening from stupidity into self-recrimination. Cara and I had spent five years building a beautiful post and beam house on a Quebec lake not far from Ottawa. It really was spectacular, twice featured in the full-page home section of the *Ottawa Citizen* newspaper, possibly a first. Building had been stressful. It was September, and as educators, we were insanely preoccupied with the business of work and life. Though the house had been the dream, with too little time and money, we craved relief from it. The real estate market was very low, so selling with not an option. We decided to rent for a year or so and forget. A couple answered my ad and were ecstatic about the beauty of the house evident from posted photos. The fact that they agreed to a long-term lease sight unseen should have been my first clue. They arrived at 7 a.m., two hours early, and being confused and trusting, I gave them the key to the house with the understanding that I would join them later in the day before any final commitment was made.

As I drove up to the meet the couple, I was aware of unease that I could not define. And with a thousand September details cluttering my brain, I was not really trying to coax unease into focus. As I cruised along a slow rise towards the Gatineau Hills with Tim Horton's coming into view, clutter and unease crystallized into certainty and dread. This precise moment is one of the clearest moments of my life, still punctuated by regret, and in concert with Doug's self-assessing thoughts of *How could I be so stupid*! The couple were professional grifters who proceeded to lock us out of our house, throw out our personal effects, attempt to charge $30,000 in our name from various department stores, and claim to be victims to the police and justice system. And inexplicably, what you learn is, the police and justice system are no more useful or sympathetic to you than to those they wistfully acknowledge are the crooks. They did offer the sage advice that we should inform our insurance company, who promptly cancelled our house insurance. The couple claimed they were not leaving, with a veiled threat that if they were forced out, they might leave our house in ashes.

Dealing with the grifters took several months, many thousands of dollars, and something of us that can never fully be recovered. We learned much, stuck together, and won against the odds to the extent it is possible to win. Memory of winning is tainted by a version of our diminished selves, which while evoking compassion for others is oddly hard to apply to self.

The all-consuming flames of Christmas 2006 have damped down into mere scorching embers of a past that was to have liberated Doug but instead placed him in prison without parole. In 15 years he has not had a night of sleep without the aid of sleeping pills. When he was able to function at all, he threw himself into work, which he says saved him. Good thing, he says dispassionately, because with the debt he has incurred, he will have to work until he dies. No joke implied.

There is something else he threw himself into that a lesser man could not have done. Even in his diminished, humiliated state of mind, without resources or support, Doug decided he had to pursue the scam artists to the ends of the earth. Doug had lost $850,000, had been informed that getting any of his money back was highly unlikely, and yet he chose a path that would ratchet up further his staggering debt. Why? Many would ask and still do. Doug reasoned that he had been cheated out of love, but he was not going to be cheated out of justice. He'd lost all of his possessions and most of himself, but he had just enough residue stuff left to fight back—and this the fraudsters had not seen and Doug did not know of himself until presented with a diminished version of himself that required he act from his residual higher self.

By now Doug's story is all over the media, to his everlasting shame, and though there is some sympathy, there is no real help. There are no go-fund-me campaigns, his legal options are limited, and the possibility of getting his money back, non-existent. Some people let it be known that he got what he deserved for being so gullible, stupid, naive, take your pick, and Doug agrees and is much harder on himself than any of those who condemn.

But whatever else Doug is, he is not weak. He steels himself to pursue justice in a legal system that disadvantages the victim, that will not give him satisfaction or happiness, but which has to be done in order to be able to look himself in the mirror. There are a few people in the persecutor's office who are helpful, but in law as in life, Doug learns he is alone. Doug is maybe one in one hundred who are willing to pursue justice in consideration of the abysmal odds, but predictable as his life has been in many ways, when faced with a crisis, he is his own man.

Though it takes years, Doug wins his case against both fraudsters. The end result of winning is why people do not do what Doug did regardless of the principle and personal integrity involved. After years of stress, legal minefields, and dead ends, the final tally of Doug's winning carnage is as follows: Danovan comes from Jamaica to Canada, not to face his fraud charges but because he needs medical treatment. While here he pleads guilty to conspiracy to commit fraud and gets a conditional sentence of 18 months under house arrest but no jail time to be served. Danovan's only defence in his non-defence was his claim that he was too busy being a coke dealer to have been concerned with petty fraud. For Doug's civil victory he received 18 100-dollar monthly payments for a total of $1,800 dollars.

Dee eventually pleads guilty of conspiracy to commit fraud and gets a sentence of three years, only serving 18 months before being freed on parole. In civil court, Doug received a symbolic payment of $3,000 before she successfully declared bankruptcy. For both cases, Doug pursued and did get a restitution order against the fraudsters, but in Ontario civil orders are up to the complainant to enforce. Good luck with that. In the end, the money ledger total read $4,800 received against a total of $850,000 stolen, plus over half a million in legal fees, for a blistering sum of $1.4 million lost. Doug has many, many regrets, but he does not regret wrestling this legal nightmare to the ground. That takes guts. And courage.

His reason for proceeding eyes wide open after being taken eyes completely shut—he wanted to make sure this never happens to anyone else. That simple, that sincere, a sacrifice, that being the type of guy Doug is. One might think naive guy naively thinking the money is coming back once he gets a restitution order, but no, part of Doug's half million-dollar legal output was used to pay an auditing firm to find where the money went and determine if any might be salvageable. Apart from tracking the money to Jamaica, the auditing firm came up empty.

Maybe Doug is, as some think, the stupidest person on earth for falling for the fraudsters. But if so, he may also have set a world record for integrity for the sacrifice he made to get even a modicum of justice. Which I suggest to Doug, which he bats away, which I understand once I ask him if he has been able to forgive himself. Big intake of breath, and he answers simply, "Not yet. Maybe someday." The fact that he has not been able to make things right with his sister regarding the will, though he bore no legal responsibility, is a sore point for which forgiveness is not possible. Doug's standard for forgiveness requires doing things right, rather than simply intending.

I suggest to Doug that his mother would likely have forgiven him long ago. Then I ask, What would she do if she suddenly appeared to you right now? He pauses, laughs, and says, "She would bawl me out for about 15 minutes and then give me a big hug." Most of all, Doug says that today he struggles with not being reconciled to his sister, whom he loves, but she will not speak to him. For a guy who can't forgive himself, it makes sense that he doesn't blame her for 15 years of continued estrangement.

I understand why Doug had to pursue the fraudsters to the ends of the earth. He knew that if he did not they would live to commit fraud another day, and many more after that. But there was something else. Doug chose his perilous path, which could not have been easy, even before his folly was exposed. Perhaps his deliberate choice was equal parts delusion and determination in the spirit of James Joyce's greatest story, *The Dead*. "Better pass boldly into that other world, in the full glory of some passion, than fade and wither dismally with age."[17]

When he described his relationship with Dee, he said that she represented the worst and best of times, the heights of great love and the depths of despair. Though he knows that she did not love him, he did not say, even after 15 years of torment, that what he had thought was love was not. I waited and wondered if he meant what he had said. To my surprise he did not recant, which puzzled me. Then it occurred to me that the love he once felt was actual love, even if misdirected, and cannot be appropriated or reassigned to some other lesser emotion. It was not merely infatuation; it was not only sexual attraction; it was love, if only for a historical heartbeat that occupied a space in Doug that he only knew existed for having experienced its soul-gripping tentacles. True, Doug needed to bring Dee to justice for altruistic reasons. But there was also that pervasive, undeniable need to make real not only what happened to him but also what he felt. He loved once, not wisely, but it was love and can't be denied. That was something.

Much of meaning comes down to love, one and indivisible. It is what is left after everything else is lost. Love remains, even if one's lover does not. We love those who do not love us back. Love is filled with should nots, but who we love is not always for us to decide. But loving in the absence of love is painful, cruel even. It is the phantom limb, a stillborn self-inflicted psychic wound that permeates our half-wakeful dreams. We cannot forget and vaguely wonder, Where does unrequited, unexpressed, never acknowledged love go?

I was brought up on a fire and brimstone version of hell. Like most kids I had nightmares about burning in hell in perpetuity. The concept of being forever consumed by flames is fairly incomprehensible to a kid of any age. In my later teens,

---

17. James Joyce, *The Dead* (Claremount: Coyote Canyon Press, 2008), 69.

I read Christopher Marlowe's *Dr. Faustus* and was fascinated by the concept of hell not as fire and brimstone but as the state that exists in the absence of God—or as a contemporary concept, the persistent hollow echo that is our life in the absence of love.

I believe that God exists in communion with whoever is placed on our path. It is that simple. In rare instances that person will be someone we love, and we may love or be loved for reasons beyond our control. For all the reasons not to love, and they are many, we cannot help but let love in sometimes, and our sometimes are not necessarily wise.

If life is the nihilistic version towards which the world is tilting, Doug, the existence of love, and all of us are in trouble. But if each of us is of spiritual origin, life is effervescent wonder, not material-world predictability, and love, even misplaced as it may be, is a repudiation of brute force determination. If God is, Doug will transcend his first failed love for the realization of his heart's desire, which really wasn't about her anyway. For his all too human failings, Doug, the unrequited, is lovable and is loved.

Chapter Twelve

"FOLLOW THE ARGUMENT WHEREVER IT LEADS"

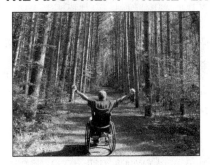

*"Miracles are a retelling in small letters of the very same story
which is written across the whole world in letters
too large for some of us to see."*

C. S. Lewis, writer, lay theologian, academic (1898–1963)

It isn't only the phenomenon of working anthropic impossibility in our lonely speck of the universe, and it isn't only the singular existence of life on same obscure piece of real estate that gives pause. Every day we experience beauty, the conscious achievement of mysterious human endeavour, and rarely do we conclude it's just science. I don't hear atheists reducing their favourite art or music down to mere sensory perception. People—atheist and materialists equally—talk in rapturous ways about what they consider beautiful, even using words such as "spiritual" to describe the experience of beauty without seeing any contradiction with their beliefs. But surely a spiritual experience is not possible for a collection of temporary living cells interacting before the cruel and *natural* end of our existence. That would not be beauty; that would be delusion.

What, then, is beauty? What can possibly inspire awe in response to beauty if we are simply biological entities without intention? A couple of years ago, I arrived at the Cologne train station while going to attend a conference. I knew Cologne had a cathedral worth visiting, but I was not prepared for the human-made wonder that towers directly over the square as one exits the station. I have to admit that this cathedral was particularly appealing to me because of my lifelong fascination with antique stained glass. Depending on your source, the Cologne Cathedral has up to ten kilometres of exquisite stained-glass panels, some dating back to the twelfth century.

It took 632 years to construct the cathedral, so whoever made the decision to build knew that they would never live to see its completion, however well building progressed. Makes you wonder. How were people ever able to commit their lives and resources to pay forward such spiritual intention, particularly of this magnitude, if survival and self-interest are the currency of existence?

Richard Dawkins objects to the waste of resources spent on cathedrals—naively assuming that money not squandered on buildings would have gone directly to the poor. The essence and hence value of a cathedral cannot be reduced to stone and mortar. Standing, looking up into the heights of the Cologne Cathedral—sculptured stone, carved wood, stained glass images depicting the history of Christianity—I noticed that even people who do not appreciate the significance of the artwork, who do not usually visit churches, who do not believe in God, visit quietly, all habitual protest temporarily laid aside, just standing, suspended, in awe (perhaps proven by the fact that no one dared punctuate and deflate the experience of awe by saying *awesome*).

Still, as the good Professor Dawkins floats along the corridors of Oxford University or walks the streets of said town, does he disparage all the beautiful buildings? Does the wasted architecture of the Christian world stand alone, or does it also represent the institutions that directly flowed from it, such as democracy, our justice system, and capitalism? Socialists deride the oppressive nature of capitalism, perhaps forgetting that capitalism created wealth where little existed, and there is nothing to equitably redistribute if nothing is created.

All human rights bodies and democratic constitutions, acts, and legislation are the imperfect product of the Judeo-Christian tradition, whose most profound and taken-for-granted feature is the radical shift towards—yes, including, but not limited to—the sanctity of the individual. It is ironic to the point of absurdity that progressive movers and shakers demonize Christianity because its version of human worth includes the unborn and not yet dead, the sanctity of life being its core principle. It is true that the introduction of the notion of *soul* into rights thinking complicates advocates' primacy of choice premise, but the possibility of life after material obliteration shouldn't be too threatening.

Dawkins saves his weakest argument for his brief explanation of consciousness. Perhaps nothing in this universe—we are not going with the multiverse theory—presents more immediate and palpable proof of God than the existence of consciousness. This claim is most often dismissed as proof of a human-centric non-scientific irrational fantasy, but for subversives who have chosen not to be overwhelmed by the tribe (Nietzsche), the existence of consciousness is not only a self-evident truth; it is the vehicle by which the physical and spiritual worlds come together and the means by which revelation becomes possible. And if Nietzsche's advice is not sufficiently old enough to evoke wisdom, a similar take on the necessity of separating from the mob comes from Marcus Aurelius (AD 121–180): "The object of life is not to be on the side of the majority, but to escape finding oneself in the ranks of the insane."

Dawkins dismisses the miracle of consciousness as nothing more than an appropriate response to nature, a natural piece of evolution—bearing in mind that his version of natural selection requires that all things happen without intention—and in no way is consciousness outside the jurisdiction of scientific materialism. He admits that consciousness represents another of his infamous scientific "gaps," but of course, *gap* is code for temporary stop-gap until science solves all mysteries, reducing everything to a version of Darwinian selection—just in case anyone doubts that plain facts rule. There is no transcendent purpose in life, so don't look for it in the intricacies of how everything fits together and maintains a universal harmonious heartbeat. Lack of intention is actually called *chaos*; the obvious all-pervasive and astonishing evidence of intricate harmony everywhere can only come from intention, and to derive harmony from chaos is the ultimate oxymoron.

Consciousness may be of our organic brain, but it is far more than grey matter. In scientific materialist thinking consciousness is merely an explanation of the far more limited, mechanical poor cousin called the brain, which is to say biology cannot and will never explain essence. The individual mind, where consciousness actually resides, cannot be accessed by science—our thinking, perceptions, memory, are all our own. Even what we choose to reveal to those we care for is very limited, impossible for many, and hence the reason for and name of this book.

And yet. In addition to our fantastical common experience of consciousness, there exists a universal higher version, what Buddhists call the continually residing mind. For some few, there is communion within an elevated, transcendental state of mind. I believe that achieving this state is possible because I have met people who definitely have an aura of spiritually that I most definitely lack. I can't prove it, but I have felt it in some very few others along my path.

The concept of consciousness as communal rather the separate shards of impersonal experience is neither original nor new. In an ancient text, consciousness as unified and personal is articulated in a manner that should make modern guru claimants of the same recoil with unoriginality, or with consistency to the text, or at least admit that it is a long-held understanding that consciousness is shared. This philosophy, called theistic monism, postulates,

> The only word in English to denote a completely unbounded consciousness being is "God." Thus, all sentient beings, seen and unseen, are simply different forms of one divine Consciousness, which looks out at the universe that is its own body through uncountable pairs of eyes. To make

it personal: you are not separate from God/dess and never have been. Indeed, you are the very means by which She knows Herself.[18]

Thinking is not what we do because we are physical beings; rather, we exercise this unexplainable phenomenon despite being animals in the material world. The ability to think, transcending time and place, the experience of love, compassion, and altruism are what makes us human, not that we can stand and speak. Modern nihilists seek to reduce our human-centric purpose into nothing and, in the non-spiritual spirit of equity, have us understand that we are just biology, no better or worse than any other living thing. As a dog guy, I can honestly claim that this thought has some appeal, but it just isn't true. We have singular attributes for a reason, and no amount of material-world thinking will ever get to the essence of our humanity.

To this point, I invoke Anthony Flew in *There Is a God*, citing his exemplar of science and logic, quantum physics pioneer Erwin Schrodinger:

> The scientific picture of the world around me is very deficient. It gives me a lot of factual information, puts all our experiences in a magnificently consistent order, but is ghastly silent about all that is really near to our heart, that really matters to us. It cannot tell a word about the sensation of red and blue, bitter and sweet, feelings of delight and sorrow. It knows nothing of beauty and ugly, good and bad, God and eternity. Science sometimes pretends to answer questions in these domains, but the answers are very often so silly that we are not inclined to take them seriously ... If its world picture does not even include beauty, delight, sorrow, if personality is cut out of it by agreement, how should it contain the most sublime idea that presents itself to the human mind?[19]

If you take God out of the equation, if you refuse to do as Anthony Flew did for 50 years and follow the argument wherever it takes you, then you have given yourself permission for vacuous speculation in place of logic and empirical evidence. Many of us are intimidated by scientists and academics in general because of their expertise. So it is refreshing to find experts whose expertise includes wonder, not only for what is glimpsed—for knowing much is to know little—but for what is unknown, for what lies completely outside of one's discipline and what may be, in an empirical sense, unknowable. The best in their fields tend to maintain a childish curiosity, which ensures that what is discovered remains about the researched topic and not the researcher.

If God is the reality that created the anthropic components, accounting for our origin and continued existence every second of all time, if all the laws of science have been ordered to draw incomprehensible perfection out of chaos; if this beauty,

---

18. Christopher D. Wallis, *The Recognition Sutras: Illuminating a 1,000-Year-Old Spiritual Masterpiece* (Chicago: Mattamayura Press, Independent Publishing Group, 2017), 324–5.
19. Flew, *There is a God*, 105.

grace, and precision gives you polite pause before accepting Dawkins's probability model (basically, humans must have won the biggest, most unlikely, lottery of all time); and if you ache for a more reasonable and satisfying answer to our existence than deeply flawed and nihilistic presumptions, give yourself permission to doubt the wisdom of rock-star Dawkins. Sure, doubt God, but keep an open mind, including finding elements of truth in your own soaring senses.

A modern nihilistic premise is that religion is oppressive, and anything that promotes individual choice is progressive. The word *progressive* is used today to denote membership in a club/tribe you want to/have to belong to. There exists a social expectation in this age of intolerance for limited thinking and narrow conformity. Moderns practice narrowness for failing to see that there are those, many actually, who know much who are neither wholly empirical nor credentialed. The examined life requires the persistent use of critical thinking, especially as applied to an evaluation of ideological or borrowed thinking. The modern unexamined life does not seek truth but to be right.

And being right can close the mind of a genius, while humility can kick open the door to revelation. Northrop Frye was arguably the greatest literary critic of his era until his death in 1991. His long night of doubt into submission came late in life with the advent of his wife's death. He was inconsolable and could not find solace in God, revealing a little-known fact that though he was an ordained Anglican minister for 50 years, he never believed in God. It is my view that Frye's articulation of grief from the heart is greater than his most important academic work. *The Great Code*, 1982, examines the Bible as literature, analyzing the archetypal and mythological heritage of Western civilization, and is unprecedented in the world of literary criticism.

Yet the great man could not move beyond grief; that is, he could not reconcile himself to the thought that the essence of his wife and all she had meant to him had simply been cells that once lived and were now dead. Although he could not proclaim belief in God in a positive sense, the revelation that his wife's essence was more than cells that temporarily lived was stronger than his long-held atheism, and therefore he fashioned, with the application of logic, what he called a negative faith. I have always found Northrop's revelation to be a very satisfying story of faith because it comes from such an unlikely source. And as a source infused with doubt and humility, without the prevalence of intellectual bias, it speaks equally to personal and shared experience.

Northrop's great intellectual engine failed him until he was forced to go to a less intellectual, less resistant, higher place. For all his intellectual understanding of the Bible as the narrative code of our civilization, he remained willfully blind to essence until he glimpsed the spiritual dimension of the one he loved. Frye's concept of negative faith is both a proclamation of faith—to accept that his wife's death has meaning changes everything—and resignation to the folly of living life exclusively from the perch of great intellectual distance. Humility over hubris in a heartbeat.

Towards the end of *The God Delusion*, Dawkins fashions the atheist life as noble, of doing good deeds without heavenly reward and bravely facing death without need for the mushy sedative of religion to dull the senses. To anyone who has loved another human being, Dawkins's self-congratulatory eulogy is disingenuous, cold comfort at best, and to anyone who has loved deeply, its repudiation of hallowed existence rings hollow.

But in the final pages, Dawkins's anticipated epiphanic victory of atheism over deism is oddly inspiring—that is, for spiritual subversives who have not yet been overwhelmed by the tribe. Dawkins makes the point that rocks and other material world matter are mostly just space, or more than 99.999… percent empty. Okay, difficult concept to comprehend, but we knew that. Then he says, try this exercise. Think back to your most vivid memory, when you were young, recalling the plethora of sensory details that pervades strong memory. He says you will remember well because you were there, after all. But then he says, here's the kicker: the you that exists, sitting remembering in this moment, hasn't a single atom in common with the former you who experienced the details being recalled. Which raises the question, if in a historic heartbeat we are emptied of our former material-world selves (whose atomic content is primarily space), even as we remain connected by memory, what is a human being? If we lose the material or human aspect of *human* being through atom exchange and death, we are left with *being*, self-evidenced by consciousness, that remains as the essence of life. Thank you, Doctor.

Flew and Frye did not finally submit because of weakness; their acknowledgement of a spiritual life was not due to age or infirmity. Both great intellects were disinclined towards faith but at least did not rebuke wisdom. Flew's conversion without faith, Frye's negative version of faith, and Dawkins's unwavering faith in himself make for interesting reading from among the intellectual titans of the modern age. Which is to say, intellect will not necessarily serve you well and can quite possibly work to your objective detriment when it comes to a consideration of faith. Faith may be *the* necessary ingredient to filling in between what is known and what is knowable in logic and in science. Faith is a sort of God particle, glue in an uncertain world, as we piece together an incomplete narrative that does not end with the certainty of despair and death.

In this sense, a necessary ingredient to having faith is searching for it. Not finding faith may be the gap that exists until we get there. The holding of faith may be life's greatest challenge. My faith is precarious at best, so I am on thin ice. But there may be something that helps in Frye's and Flew's circuitous route to conceding to God. Even Dawkins's resistance to following wherever the argument leads is instructive and might lead people to re-examine the emptiness of his message, especially as he ends *The God Delusion* indulging in pop psychology. Dawkins likens having faith in God to a child having an imaginary friend. Far from disparaging childhood, I suspect that faith has much to do with the marriage of childhood wonder to the wisdom of the ages. From David Bentley Hart's book, the epiphany moment, "wisdom is the recovery of innocence at the end of experience."[20]

Even Albert Einstein, the twentieth century's most accomplished scientist, never lost perspective on the non-scientific elemental origin of human drive. "I have no special talent. I am only passionately curious." Dawkins tells us that we must discard imaginary friends and grow up. But to achieve this point of maturation the adult must embrace the death culture of nihilism. To which I say, embrace wonder, practice openness, search for wisdom, and refuse to grow up.

Heretic as I may be to the glory of science, remember that even Stephen Hawking says that fidelity to materialism logically leads to the greater problem and remaining question of "What is it that breathes fire into equations and makes a universe for them to describe?" Perhaps more pointed questions for human beings wrestling with the puzzle of consciousness are these: What do we do with our overwhelming feelings of love, regret, loss, despair, and joy and the wellspring of self-evident truths that modernity denies or denies has meaning? Is the curse of consciousness—the inarticulate speech of our heart—the closing off of childhood wonder and hard-won wisdom, or can it be a portal to the soul, breaking through materialism, ignorance, and the social ennui of modernity?

I wrote *Lament for Spilt Porter* from instinct and fear, borrowing a bit of my dad's maverick logic and with generous infusions of childish wonder leading to a modicum of faith for which I felt and feel lacking but that at least has placed me outside of the creeping black hole of nihilism. I pondered and wrote so as not to despair. Some, perhaps many, assume that those are the very ingredients that would make me ripe for believing what I want to believe and writing a self-justifying, anti-evidence-based version of faith.

But here's the thing—my dad's skepticism has made it more difficult for me to stop questioning and have faith than to simply believe and accept, well, anything. Still, over time, in applying skepticism to the evidence for and against God's existence, I've been surprised. Ultimately, an intangible rubric of faith matters most, but for those searching for something they can grasp, weigh, and dispassionately ponder, it turns out that there is an impressive, empirical, and growing body of scientific literature that builds towards the logic of God.

For those whose faces curl into an expression equivalent to biting into a sour lemon at the mention of faith, consider this. An emerging belief system is that the universe made itself (Lawrence Kraus, in *A Universe from Nothing*, says it all); the world evolved on its own with the laws of physics existing without much thought to causation; physical reality is all there is; and spirituality has been delegitimized by the dogma and deeds of the dominant theistic religions. In this sense, scientific endeavour is losing its tradition of empirical detachment, which is the basis of its credibility. And it is no wonder. People are increasingly reading, capitulating, parking

20. David Bentley Hart, *The Experience of God: Being, Consciousness, Bliss* (New Haven and London: Yale University Press, 2013), 331.

their faith in materialist emissaries as portals to understanding science and using this narrow view to interpret the very nature and origin of our existence.

Though Dawkins's work calls for the end of religious superstition, a strict and closed version of scientific materialism is simply science devoid of reason. Interestingly, I found an opposing view in the surprisingly relevant writings of Pope John Paul II. *Faith and Reason* characterizes modernity as having devolved into a culture of death.[21] The astonishing thing about *Faith and Reason*, consistent with John Paul's writings and world view, is not his recitation of Catholic orthodoxy but rather his progressive, perhaps postmodern, belief that reason and faith cannot be separated and that religion can turn into superstition if it cuts itself off from reason. Hm, turns out the supposed defender of traditional close-minded religious oppression is more open to science and reason than many of his credentialed opponents.

It seems odd, and scientific materialism appears lacking when it attempts to explain non-material phenomenon such causation, origin, and meaning. There is nothing wrong with taking discussion of science to philosophical speculation—in fact, a central argument I want to emphasize is that new discoveries in science logically and increasingly lead to informed speculation about events that cannot be fully or even partially explained by science and therefore beg for non-material answers—that is, the existence of God. This point and John Paul II's central point are critical. Faith is not fantasy or willful thinking; it is seeing a link between what our senses tell us—aided by empirical evidence—and what we sense to be true. And what we sense to be true employs intellect, instinct, and all our human and spiritual resources; in other words, it seeks synthesis where through the cascading waters of life's complexities it exists.

It is easy to deny or forget that all societies, cultures, and indigenous peoples, until this narrow breath of time in which we now live, believed that another world outside of or in addition to or eclipsing the material world exists. Perhaps hard to get our heads around, but people throughout time took spiritual existence beyond our ability to see to be a self-evident truth, just as we believe in the limited evidence of our own narrow vision today. We have regressed.

And why do we repress and disparage impersonal archetypal belief as well as personal self-evidence of transcendent truth for the death cult of modern thought? Quite simply, we have lost faith in the strength, the wisdom, and even the existence of our mind. Consciousness is no longer regarded as the vehicle to transcend, connect, and most significantly confirm our singular existence but rather is equated with grey matter function, with thinking and exercising of free will relegated to the lowly determinism of utilitarian neurons. As Michael Behe ponders in his astonishing critique of our highly flawed capitulation to all things Darwin, "How did science—the very discipline we use to understand the physical world—

---

21. John Paul II, *Fides et Ratio: On the Relationship Between Faith and Reason* (Boston: Pauline Books and Media, 1998).

get to the bizarre point where some otherwise very smart people use it to deny the existence of the mind?"[22]

Scientists who are not open to following Flew's argument wherever it takes them have shielded their eyes from the inconvenient truth of modern science, and this is especially true of the last 20 or 30 years. And yes, I am saying the following: Anthony Flew, 50 years an atheist, who changed his mind on the basis of evidence leading to philosophical reasoning; Pope John Paul II, 27 years a pope, from the point of view of reason being *the* necessary ingredient to having and holding faith; and modern scientists who are actually aware of and willing to follow the dispassionate findings of their discipline do not all share an allegiance to a subjective argument that uses science to support a predetermined bias but rather arrive at a common view based on the indisputable facts of logic and science. I know many people would laugh at the notion of the good Doctor Dawkins being bested for scientific objectivity by the bad Pope Paul, and yet that is where the evidence leads. Their respective works are worth reading with both skepticism and an open mind.

• • •

... including self-evident truths ...

With all our inglorious fakery, we pretend to know. From the cradle to the grave. We are distracted, comforted into denial, bolstered by modernity. Modernity tell us what we need to know and assures us that we do know, always. Google gives us instant facts. We have instant access to all that is known. With a few clicks we are privy to the known without having to know. It appears on our screen for an instant.

History is out of fashion; wisdom is for old people; God is dead. The unknowns are merely details to be soon worked out or discovered by science, posted for instant access in the near, modern, and therefore better future.

Still, deep down we only know we do not know. We are informed by fear. We are not fearful because we are weak; we are weak because we deny fear. Life, a life well-lived, in addition to everything else is to admit to fear. We fear the limited we do know—that we are naked and exposed, that we are alone. Gazing up at the stars, we feel our insignificance in the face of the physical universe. Overwhelming, except for the distinct possibility that God is.

God is not ordinary. If God *is*, then every facet of life at all times is extraordinary. If God isn't, then every facet of ordinary life is extraordinarily cruel, with meaningless pain and loss adding insult to the injury of our foreknowledge of personal obliteration. It has never been true that the revelation of God is revealed to us in our ordinary lives; that is, revelation only occurs to those who can exit the willful blindness of ordinary existence and see the *it* that God is.

The extraordinary of ordinary that we have to embrace exists in Joan Osborne's epiphany line from "One of Us": "What if God was one of us; Just a slob like one of us." It is no coincidence that materialism has come to fruition in the modern world; the distractions are endless, and if God isn't, we need to be distracted from

---

22. Behe, *Darwin Devolves*, 258.

purposeless life and the inevitably of death. If God is, one has to radically and deliberately alter one's view of life to see beyond the faux extraordinary of distraction to the authentic extraordinary of ordinary everyday life. God and his failure to reveal himself and convince us is not the problem. We are the problem. We, fully endowed with the expansive potential of consciousness—the Gran Telescope Canarias, the world's biggest telescope equivalent—are closing our collective eyes.

So, the ordinary and easy life we all seem to desire may be our greatest limitation to seeing God. And the marginalized people we shun or exclude and the tendency towards angst and wonder that we discourage or kill out of fidelity to bland may be where we have most to learn, may explain why most of us do not learn, why modernity is winning. Turns out, we've been looking for love in all the wrong places.

As a child in the boredom of school and church I pondered the wonder of the stars, the mystery of what it is to be human, and the supreme unlikelihood of our existence. Once curiosity is forged, we have to find a way to sustain it, our willful and subversive resistance to distraction and bland. Oddly, this opportunity for openness can present itself in the form of painful circumstances, the experience of extremity, and resistance to being overwhelmed by the tribe. More odd, because we do not seek painful circumstances; we do not easily see opportunity for growth in tragedy. Oddest yet, because the wistful day-dreaming refusal to embrace distraction that keeps us from pondering the universe and our place in it is regarded as wasting time. To never have a thought about our origin and purpose is totally acceptable today as long as we are willing to virtue signal nonthinking appropriate and abstract causes within a very narrow range of possibility.

Growing up we had expectations related to church, school, and family but not restrictions to thinking, no limiting concern for self-esteem, no ideologies and distractions of any kind. Under strict Catholic rules, and in a family of nine, we were free to think, to know at least that this one little life was not about any one of us. Following rules and being ruled are not the same thing. The mind, awareness in consciousness, including and especially awareness of our spiritual nature, is freedom, a freedom that nihilists want us to freely give up.

As a kid, I'd sit at my parents' kitchen table among people, but silent and just outside of social interaction. The memory of our kitchen table is also fused with the searing impression of my dad's accident during the war, of his lifetime of immobility, of his inability to express his pain, of our family's difficulty connecting with each other, our family's inarticulate speech of the heart. My metaphoric parents' kitchen table from which I seek solitude, contemplate, and listen is sought in perpetual movement, and in the obvious reaction to my father's immobility, I am my father's son. Thirty years a competitive distance runner, 30 years working with persons with disabilities, and in more recent, softer times, long walks, hikes, still running, kayaking, long, spontaneous car drives, always forward movement, searching for something towards a finish line I will never cross—at least not in this lifetime— distracting from distraction, something there, something important, can't quite see it, still out of focus even at times of rare revelation, vaguely sensing the blue linoleum kitchen table with the stainless steel legs, unsure if I am going forward or backwards, and unconcerned about direction as long as I keep moving. If there is any poetry to my motion it is in waiting for I know not what but knowing it will come. Or perhaps I'm simply trying to live by an Albert Einstein axiom: "Life is like riding a bicycle. To keep your balance, you must keep moving."

Though I am, have always been, a searcher, I am also an occasional denier. And by that I mean beyond the skepticism and doubt of a self-described maverick. Because, and I hate to admit, fused to maverick is modern man. I was confronted with this sad fact in recent times. For years on an occasional basis we have had the hall lights in our house at three locations inexplicably go on or off. Explicable perhaps because it is a 100-year-old house; inexplicable perhaps because the entire house was rewired ten years ago. We have jokingly said that this must be Mom's way of reminding us that she is still around, so confirmation that there is life after death.

During Christmas Day dinner two years ago, the chandelier in the dining room went off twice in the space of five minutes, which had never happened before and has never since. Oh, Mom again, we joked, and we forgot about. Two weeks later, I was at work on a brilliantly beautiful winter day that was perfect for skating on our city's renowned eight kilometre canal. I decided to take a rare and hurried noontime skate but needed to travel home from work to get my skates and clothes—a bit of an inconvenience, but my house is near the university, and both locations are within easy walking distance of the canal.

I needed to pull together clothes for cold weather and hurried upstairs to the chest of drawers in my bedroom. I opened the top sock drawer and stood momentarily trying to decide what I needed, even as a selection of the required clothing stared me in the face. My mind was hurried and distracted, 100 percent grounded or limited by material-world preoccupation. Immediately over top my sock drawer is our stereo receiver, and during my moment of suspended preoccupation, the radio loudly came on, the panel lit up, and classical music filled the house.

Never before or since has this happened to any of us, and certainly not while at the exact moment of standing inches away from the stereo in a large empty house. What did I do? I snapped off the power, without considering how it had come on, turned around, and walked over to get something, but since I did not need anything in that direction, I simply stopped and stood still. I suppressed what had happened and what it might mean for a lazy, dismissive *whatever,* our collective modern defence against any potential material-world intrusion. Even so, I am not saying that I denied an obvious visitation from my dearly departed Mom, because I just don't know. What I am saying is that whatever it was, at that moment I was closed to possibility, I was blind to potential, I was a thoroughly modern man. Not knowing while still wondering in life is life; faux knowing and denying in life is death in advance of the fact.

Which brings us back to Peter's statement, the one that both disturbs and matters most, provokes and can serve to enhance or undermine equilibrium, our sense of normalcy, and quite possibly, faith: Even if God does exist, he isn't interested in me.

Peter's words, especially the particular and deliberate phrasing he used, had surprised me, but they really should not have. Leading up to his blunt assessment of God, Peter had expressed openness to the question of God's existence. That discussion had been mostly about my recently digested scientific readings, and Peter had agreed that there was merit in my reasoning. Our conversation had been about the concept, logic, and evidence that supported the existence of an impersonal God, and Peter had finally and simply responded to his very personal experience of 45 years as a quadriplegic, a response anyone might easily come to after four minutes of the same.

Still, since there actually is no meaning outside of our connection to others, it is perhaps less an indulgence than a responsibility that we actively engage with others, that we seek commonality in the seemingly most distant human experience from our own. The problem of pain seems to be the place of greatest resistance to faith, and for good reason, but at least we have this: whatever life's trajectory, however rich or poor, tragic or lucky, our experience, our lives all come to the same elemental trifecta. For all the beauty and richness of living, we *all* experience pain, loss, and death.

Which is not to say all experience is equal. Painful experience may or may not make it more difficult to believe in a personal relationship with God, but God's existence is not based on whether or not we believe. Nor does the numbing effect of pain prove there is no purpose in it. If God is, there is purpose in pain. If there is purpose in pain—and obviously the experience of pain is very uneven—then it stands to reason that those who experience disproportionately more pain have a greater claim to its purpose. The fact that we cannot see what the purpose could possibly be does not mean the purpose is not there, since we can neither see nor would ever willingly choose pain and how is it allocated. Sure, according to materialists everything is luck, karma, stuff that just happens, but these mindless majority explanations explain nothing.

Peter's statement about a personal God was particularly disturbing because it had been worming its way through my brain long before I met him, back to a moment when I was about 10 years old. Sometime in the mid-60s, I saw a series of images in a documentary film about the liberation of Second World War concentration camps in Poland. The most poignant and disturbing scene: hundreds of skeletal naked bodies bulldozed into open pits, without narration or sound of any kind. Strangely, I think the silence even more than the visual images grafted on to my naked memory for its moving and poignant emptiness. How could life come to this? The innumerable rotting cadaverous remains had all been individual human beings once but utterly lacked humanity, and to my 10-year-old sensibilities the images were irreconcilable with everything I had known until that moment. My view of life has never been the same.

It has often been said that during the Holocaust many observant Jews lost their faith. Easy to understand, easy to take as fact what is often said. But in the preface to *Man's Search for Ultimate Meaning*, Victor Frankl dispenses with the assumption that faith necessarily dies with the experience of hardship, even of the most brutal nature. "The truth is that among those who actually went through the experience of Auschwitz, the number of those whose religious experience was deepened—in spite of, not because of, this experience—by far exceeds the number of those who gave up their belief."[23]

Jews, fully integrated citizens of Europe, had been subjected to the most brutal state-sponsored hate crime in history to the tune of six million individual lives lost. Families were dragged out of their homes, put on cattle cars, too crowded to sit or lie down, and forced to travel for days in this torturous state without food or water. For those who survived the deportation to Auschwitz, Treblinka, Buchenwald, or any of the dozens of death camps, upon arrival there was either instant selection for the gas chamber or the chance to be worked and starved to death as a labourer. Children, the elderly, and the most vulnerable were always selected for instant death, since they had no value as labourers.

Less well-known than the concentration camp murder machine is the more prolific Holocaust by bullets that occurred in the wake of the German assault on the Soviet Union. Operation Barbarossa, launched on June 22, 1941, remains the greatest military battle in history with approximately three million German soldiers facing an even greater number of Soviet troops. Peripheral to the central military operation was the necessity to purge the civilian population of Jews in the newly occupied territories. Hastily recruited military police units were assigned this task behind the lines of the massive armies that moved across Eastern Europe and the Ukraine into the Soviet Union.

Packaged in the guise of dispassionate duty and necessary racial cleansing, the process of killing by these police units was the epitome of impersonal. Crimes against humanity require a large and willing segment of humanity to voluntarily commit inhumane acts. City, town, and village citizens surrendered their neighbours and fellow citizens for certain murder simply because they were Jewish. Though some individuals were disgusted and resistant, the great revelation of the twentieth century was the extent to which a vendetta and mob mentality transformed average people into gleeful killers of average people they had lived beside in perfect harmony their whole lives.

The welling of dormant grievance into murder and plunder was so spontaneous and combustible in the sweep across Eastern Europe that even the Germans were surprised by the complicity of non-Germans. Perhaps the route to murder is as simple as this: "Auschwitz begins wherever someone looks at a slaughterhouse and

---

23. Viktor E. Frankl, *Man's Ultimate Search for Meaning* (New York, Basic Books, 2000), 19.

thinks: they're only animals" (Theodor W. Adorno). Historical context, recitation of past grievance, and psychological explanations contribute to understanding but are not enough. The history of evil is beyond the study of history.

The killing ritual was eerily similar from town to town, mass murder conducted with an attempt at military precision. Victims were forced from their homes into a central gathering spot in their town, a place of familiarity somewhere nearby, inconspicuous, though not completely unknown. Hundreds or thousands were then marched from the noise and distraction of their town or village to a quiet space, perhaps into the forest, but not necessarily secluded or hidden from observation. The place of execution had been prepared, with a fresh pit dug to a size necessary to hold as many bodies as were to be murdered on that day in that particular town.

People were forced to strip completely naked and wait in a long line as the first victims were positioned along the edge of the pit, one for each soldier whose task was to perform the act of murder against a legion of victims they did not know, had not met. Bodies fell forward and were then positioned according to the sardine method—that is, lined up beside each other, head and feet in the same direction, then reversing the direction of head and feet for each layer in order to maximize the number of bodies that could fit into the pit. This was a plan, after all.

Each new recruit had to steel his nerves for his first kill. The victim is naked in all senses of the word: stripped of clothes, stripped of dignity, and stripped of humanity and any sense of its extension beyond physical existence. The recruits did not realize it, but they too were metaphorically stripped—even if cocooned in their German uniforms—of understanding, of compassion, of their souls' existence. Waiting in line, watching, hearing, and smelling death in anticipation of their own, victims were not spared from the reality of their deliberate and imminent demise. The essence of the singular person that they were had been stripped for the impersonal victim they had become.

Police units worked in long shifts; there was much work to do. The first kill might take a while as the new recruit came to terms with his required task. But getting the job done did not allow for the indulgence of hesitation, self-doubt, and conscience. The long line of stripped victims had to be managed so that a constant flow of fodder could be mowed down without losing time. If the number of Jews to be murdered on a given day was 2,500—higher than average but certainly with precedence—and if there were five killing lines—which from photos seems about right—and if each kill took one minute—which seems astonishingly quick, but we are talking about a killing machine—then, even without a break, reaching the allotted total of murders would take over eight hours.

And of course, breaks were necessary. Some victims did not strip easily or step forward to their death with German efficiency; some mothers protested the shooting of their babies; some people fell to the ground, making it difficult for recruits to take aim; and the pile of bodies directly below each lineup eventually became too high and needed to be levelled and rearranged into sardine style in order to maintain maximum pit capacity. Meanwhile, veterans drank alcohol and ensured that new recruits drank their way into becoming hard, blindly distracted, senses so dulled and corrupted by habit and drink that they were able to diminish their humanity into brutal material function.

To say that murdering at close range (recruits were to aim eight inches from the base of the skull) is corrosive to the murderer is perhaps the understatement of the turbulent twentieth century. German military planners worried about the effect of intimate, impersonal murder (perhaps the twentieth century's most horrible oxymoron) upon soldiers. Particularly worried was the man in charge of the killing machine, Heinrich Himmler. In fact, the stress on soldiers, not concern for the victims, is the main reason why the gassing factories of the concentration camps were developed—further decrease the intimacy between murderer and murder victim, and stress is proportionately reduced.

Since the Second World War, the question regarding what choice German soldiers had to resist murdering Jews has persisted. To comprehend the incomprehensible, surely the German soldiers were victims too? Perhaps in some small measure, but the relativity argument does not fit history. In Daniel Jonah Goldhagen's PhD thesis, Harvard, developed into a prize-winning book entitled *Hitler's Willing Executioners*, the question is meticulously studied for over 500 pages.

> A remarkable aspect of the transition to wholesale slaughter was how "normal" it was to the men of the Einsatzkommandos and other units that were contributing to genocide. In their post-war testimony, the killers hardly remark upon the expansion of the scope of the killing to include women, children, the aged, or to the increased size and speed of the slaughter.[24]

Though there is no normal to killing innocents, the acclimatization from doubt to willing executioner was remarkably fast and inclusive. The facts are these: generally the killing units were not staffed by hardened soldiers, for those were fighting Stalin in the Soviet Union; killer recruits were generally average Germans (most did not even belong to the Nazi party) who, though encouraged to participate in murder, were *not* forced to do so; and with the option to not kill perhaps difficult but always possible, only approximately one out of one hundred individual recruits opted to forgo murder for reassignment elsewhere.

The process of acclimation is aptly described in a letter home by a German soldier to his wife on the occasion of receiving orders to expand the shooting of men to include women and children. The soldier said that at first shooting, soldiers levelled their guns with shaky hands, but by the tenth woman or child killed, soldiers were calm and shot with a steady hand. Soon even calm was replaced by a willing

---

24. Daniel Goldhagen, *Hitler's Willing Executioners: Ordinary Germans and the Holocaust* (New York: Vintage Books, 1997), 152.

gamesmanship that had babies thrown into the air and shot for sport, no doubt to alleviate the boredom of assembly line killing. All of which raises the question: just what did soldiers think about as they bent low and levelled a gun to the back of the head of a naked, shivering five-year-old child?

Who are you and where is your personal God as you inhale and pull the trigger for the sixtieth time that day? As you witness the moment of life's departure from unique human beings and watch pathetic flesh tumble into an indistinguishable quagmire of rotting flesh, who are you? Later, upon waking at night, days or decades later, the dulling effects of alcohol gone, do you think: *My work, my life*? Even if you are able to maintain the soldierly fiction of duty to the fatherland, lying awake under the cover of darkness and hearing the silent scream that will never go away, who are you? For millions of totally exposed and innocent people, their murderer was not simply a soldier but the anti-Christ, the perverse substitute for and inversion to a personal loving God.

Tragically, to some Jews who stood at the edge of the open pit seconds before murder, God was not simply absent, but his non-intervention was proof of evil's final victory over goodness; it was proof that God had been defeated; it was witness that God was dead. History seems to validate Peter's statement about the absence of a loving God. The question is not the validity of Peter's or six million Jews' experience, for that is incontestable, but rather the validity of the conclusion that these evil acts, antithetical to any sense of justice, are evidence of God's hand.

History teaches us at every turn that there is no justice in this world, that our human expectations will always be disillusioned by what actually is. And if we adhere to the atheists' view that we are simply cells that live and die and that biology has no spiritual component, it follows that what we do in life and how we die has no purpose, and judgment of any human action is irrelevant. It is literally true in the atheists' worldview—especially since there is no view of life outside of the physical world—that the murder of a shivering, naked five-year-old standing at the edge of a mass grave in 1942 and the death of her murderer peacefully in his sleep 60 years later are no different. There is even the possibility of a perverse Darwinian view that the latter is superior to the former for its survival longevity. Even atheists overwhelmingly reject this reasoning, though it is consistent with their logic.

For anyone who has been visited upon by the ravishes of circumstance or the evil that men do, there is no satisfying argument that will alleviate personal pain. Nor is there logic in assigning the effects of circumstance and evil to God. All theistic religions have archetypal certainty about the goodness of God despite the inevitability of pain and death, which leads to a central tenet of life as struggle between the dichotomous realities of good and evil.

We accept all the good—the fact of our existence and why it is bestowed upon us—without question, but bad and evil are assigned to the presence or absence of God. In many ways, understandable, particularly for those who have faced painful extremity, but still not logical. Evil is real, God is its antithesis, and why goodness—

that is God—does not, cannot, destroy evil is the great unknowable challenge of life and death. We accept our existence without much thought to a personal origin of our unique person; we do not accept and personalize any interference to our existence, including and perhaps especially the fact of death.

The atheist has to confront this problem: if there is no God, there is nothing to judge; there is no meaning; and nothing matters, including any action committed either for good or evil, because without meaning we cannot even call an act good or evil. The theist has another problem. If there is God, our actions have meaning, and actions have consequences that can be judged as good or evil. Can we believe that God is personally indifferent to Peter? Can we believe that God personally hated or was indifferent to that five-year-old girl and then proceeded to murder her? Why is the existence of evil God's responsibility? The incomprehensible presence of evil is not the comprehensible absence of God.

The solution for the atheist is to attempt to attribute meaning to meaningless causes and heightened human experience, which must seem frivolous even to the gurus of modernity. The solution for the theist is to rid ourselves of the notion that what happens in this physical life—whether just or not—necessarily determines our spiritual life. Perhaps the evidence of pain and suffering in the absence of justice but in the presence of meaning is about the soul, independent of what our physical person desires.

Those who suffer most may do so in sacrifice for others, which may be the soul's purpose, even if at the expense of the human form it inhabits. One's personal God may exist in choosing disproportionate suffering in life—out of pure sacrifice, out of pure love—for reasons I do not necessarily like or understand or at some level even accept, except that once everything has been considered, this outlandish concept has possibility. God is improbable to many, but remember Sherlock's logic mantra that once you eliminate the impossible—which applies to the chances of anthropic components existing without intention or six million deaths in the Holocaust existing without meaning—you are left with the truth. Reuse of Sherlock may appear a leap from logic until you consider that the trifecta of pain and loss and death makes no sense as simply material world survival of the fittest coming to its natural conclusion. I may be off base and am frequently wrong, but it is true that viewed through the lens of sacrifice, loss and extremity appear much different.

Scientific materialism is antithetical to mystery. Embracing mystery that is a constant of life does not end science; rather it allows us to pursue scientific explanations with an open mind. It is a mystery why we suffer and why some suffer more than others. We cannot solve this problem, but perhaps we can stop seeing it as a problem to be solved by progressive notions of fairness. We do not have to like suffering and should always do what we can to alleviate suffering for ourselves and for others. Pain and loss, and how we conduct ourselves in the absence of knowing exactly why we suffer, may be central to our purpose in the cosmic contraction we call our life.

Our existence, sustained every second against fantastical odds, is intentional, and since that intention is not of our own origin, we are not of our own making. Seems obvious, and yet many of us live with the inward gaze, confusing our preoccupations with our purpose. And any time we doubt our purpose, all we have to do is assume the outward view. The universe and our world burst with purpose. The anthropic components maintain our unlikely equilibrium, with deliberate finetuning, if not consciously at least existing as proof of cosmic consciousness. Darwin's theory, far from demonstrating nature's mindless and brutal self-sufficiency, shows purpose to live, to thrive, and to replicate in every cell, at every moment. The wonder of Darwin's work that has been lost is that it demonstrates less survival through competition than co-operation through purpose. By logical extension, the co-operation and communion in the give and take of jostling bodies on my, your, everyone's path is our best bet for separating good from evil and discovering our personal God in the eyes of all we are privileged to encounter.

• • •

... consciousness and the articulation of a personal God

For most of us, most of the time, despite waking in the full knowledge of inevitable death, we manage to face life with a sense of purpose. Why are we not bowled over by this reality? This fact, which we generally take for granted, is really quite incredible. Collective denial doesn't explain how we are able to do this, nor does embracing the glory of atheistic purpose in transitioning from living magnificence into compost. Materialists often talk of life's mission in the pursuit of personal goals—that is, of having great purpose in the absence of any lasting purpose. And, God love 'em (but she doesn't exist, so forget that), it is a tough proposition to square purpose with fidelity to the material world that materialists are left with.

It is not human hubris but the self-evident truth of our existence revealed through consciousness that tells us we are more than compost. It may even be that solace from isolation exists in our pervasive core drive to be and do. With foreknowledge, with consciousness, why are we people not ground into depression and inertia if material death is the end of our existence? Why are the elderly often the most content of us all in the knowledge of certain imminent death? Why are people in difficult-to-impossible circumstances—whose lives are defined by struggle—often exemplars of a purpose-driven existence? Throughout human history primitive-to-civilized peoples have shared an archetypal sense of purpose based on a belief in an afterlife to follow material death. It is only very recently, in a historical heartbeat really, that the deeply personal self-evident truth of purpose based on faith has been supplanted by ideological conformity to an inward-looking modern world that repudiates the actual history of how we came to be.

Our purpose does not derive from our will. Human-centric as it seems, the universe has conspired or has been directed to provide or enhance our sense of purpose. And yes, I am shamefully human-centric because the evidence says that we are, while not the centre of the universe, the reason for its existence. And once we get over ourselves for basking in this claim, we can begin to appreciate the astonishing fact of breathing and living in this moment.

Fidelity to things outside self (the basis of my faith) and logic (in combination with but not limited to known science) is far more compelling than modern materialism. And if I might add, far more compelling than belief in self. Call it low self-esteem or being helplessly out of sync with the modern world, but I can't help thinking that even materialists must occasionally wince at the prospect of belief in self as our reason for being. Consciousness—that is, our ability to see intention and have purpose—is very much related to our place in the universe, to our singular vantage point, to our bloody-minded isolation, though not necessarily loneliness. We are alone in the universe, and we are alone for a reason.

> What several decades of research has revealed about the Earth's location within the vastness of the cosmos can be summed up in this statement: the ideal place for any kind of life as we know it turns out to be a solar system like ours, within a galaxy like the Virgo supercluster, within a super-supercluster like the Laniakea super-supercluster. In other words, we happened to live in the best, perhaps the one and only, neighbourhood that allows not only for physical life's existence but also for its enduring survival.[25]

When we gaze out at the starry night and are filled with our insignificance, maybe our interpretation is wrong. Maybe the vastness, the incomprehensible complexity, and our place in it are a reason for reverence, but not insignificance. Maybe we should appreciate our splendid isolation and contemplate our singular existence.

Which may be what the characters with character I have met in my work have to teach me. Maybe disability, isolating as it can be, has a splendid aspect allowing us to see through darkness into the light, as we do from Earth to the stars, from material distraction to spiritual meaning. Maybe location is all about perspective, from where purpose and awareness reside. Our much criticized and unfashionable tendency to be human-centric may not be a failing, may be necessary to awareness and purpose.

Our need for perspective through the portal of consciousness within the vastness of space may be where human purpose and the existence of the universe come together. For this reason, Rosenblum and Kuttner subtitle their book *Quantum Enigma* as *Physics Encounters Consciousness*. Extrapolating from Einstein's remark, in acknowledgement of the application of quantum mechanics beyond the micro into the largely unexplored macro universe, Rosenblum and Kuttner question the very nature of material-world existence. If, as quantum mechanics says, the observer or consciousness can change the behaviour of observed atoms in micro and macro levels, can consciousness affect the

---

25. Huge Ross, *Improbable Planet: How Earth Became Humanity's Home* (Grand Rapids: Baker Books), 41.

universe? Has consciousness been determining outcomes in the universe? Can consciousness have affected the universe that created it—that is, have affected a phenomenon that existed before its creation?[26]

Though consciousness is not tangible—and medically speaking, if not for its actual existence cannot be proven to be real—it is the fundamental basis of our existence; it is who we are. As Rosenblum and Kuttner postulate macro interpretations of consciousness, one cannot help but draw parallels between the vastness of the cosmos, the mystery of consciousness, and the extremity of human experience. Why extremity? If there is anything to the connection between cosmos and consciousness, it will not be revealed to the passive mind and easy life. Revelation of intention, mysteries of the universe, and the experience of extremity are forever active phenomena.

We are all in this together, and yet we live as cosmic shards of separateness. Deep down beneath distraction and denial, we disparage the unexamined life. Fundamental to the examined life is the desire to connect our life with someone else's examined life. The greatest exploration of consciousness—which surpasses the exploration of the universe—is to seek insight, transcend, and connect with the consciousness of someone else. "As the history and philosophy of science has shown in the last 150 years, when we lose the ability to recognize the work of another mind in the powerful purposeful arrangements of nature, we lose the ability to recognize even our own minds."[27]

In this sense, consciousness is less grey matter than our possibility to transcend, to connect, to realize potential. Decades earlier, the link was made between the consciousness of the intelligent observer and the natural world. "Nobel Prize winner Werner Heisenberg (1901–1976), a titan of early twentieth century physics, suggested that underlying all matter is an indivisible and unseen realm, for which he coined the term *Potentia*, and from which objects spring into existence when observed by the intelligent observer."[28] Perhaps Heisenberg's Potentia correlates to the potential of consciousness, human purpose, the realization of transcendence—what my friend Dr. John reminds me Buddhists have known for centuries—the existence of the continually residing mind. That is, each of us are among the "unaccountable pairs of eyes" that participate in consciousness as "the very means by which She knows Herself."[29]

Perhaps Bernard Haisch best articulates the unrealized potential of consciousness in an endorsement of *The Physics of God*.

It is essentially an article of faith among scientists that consciousness somehow arises in the brain and as such must be a product of evolution.

26. Rosenblum and Kuttner, *Quantum Enigma: Physics Encounters Consciousness* (USA, Oxford University Press, 2006).

27. Behe, *Darwin Devolves*, 275.

28. Selbie, *The Physics of God*, 33.

29. Wallis, *The Recognition Sutras*, 325.

This stubborn insistence that physical brain processes must be the source of consciousness will sooner or later prove to be a dead-end. What will take its place, Selbie predicts, is recognition that consciousness is the only thing that is real, is the source of the apparent physical world, and is by its nature spiritual. Once we understand that all is consciousness manifesting in different ways, a whole new worldview will open up for mankind.[30]

Our ultimate purpose may exist in pursuing the great contradiction of consciousness, its seemingly individual, locked-in nature, versus our archetypal desire to transcend and connect, to solve the mystery of our inarticulate speech of the heart. In seeking connection with whomever God places in our path, in acknowledgement of "but for the grace of God," we are in relationship with God.

Consciousness represents both our liberation and our shackles. While the sep-arateness of consciousness is a common experience, unless we have willfully closed it off, we will have insight into another's experience, moments of bliss that cannot be explained. In *Let There Be Light*, Stephen Hage argues that rather than simply having consciousness, we are *in* consciousness; that is, perhaps consciousness itself is the reality that supersedes material-world unreality, which we have access to even if we fail to access its potential most of the time.[31] In that sense, living *in* consciousness is our potential for spiritual purpose, just as an unobserved atom is potentiality unrealized until observed. We are the ultimate macro and spiritual potential achievement of quantum mechanics.

So, in answer to Peter's question/claim about the existence of a personal God, we, in relation to each other, are as close as any one of us gets in this life to a personal God. God is literally whomever God places in our path, and we are alone in order to learn how not to be. Life's purpose comes down to making connection with others, with God. Turns out they are the same thing.

---

30. Bernard Haisch, endorsement in Selbie, *The Physics of God*.
31. Stephen Hage, *Let There be Light: Physics, Philosophy and the Dimensional Structure of Consciousness* (New York: Algora Publishing, 2013).

EPILOGUE

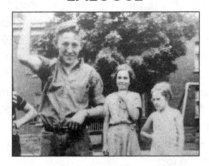

"I would love to live like a river flows, carried by the surprise of its own unfolding."

Unfinished poem, John O'Donohue, writer, philosopher, mystic

(1956–2008)

There is a photo of my dad. He stands in the middle of a group, the centre of attention, holding court as he works a lasso around his head at Gladstone Park, his neighbourhood in lower town. He is looking at the camera, an easy cocky expression on his face, and though only about 15 years old, maybe in 1936, he exudes a mischievous confidence. And in that expression, in what he exudes and the seeming fluidity of movement captured by a still photograph, lies a deep unfathomable mystery.

That moment was before; all we ever knew of Dad was after. Kids, including and especially adult kids, have a hard time seeing their parents as other than parents. But it is precisely in seeing them before, other than as parents, that recognition lies. We never saw this photo until after his death. It was a side to Dad that he buried on the day he broke his back during a storm at sea when he was 20. There is more insight into Dad in this photo of him at 15 than we learned about him, from him, during his entire life. Dad's accident contributed to the inarticulate speech of my family's heart, but looking at this photo 80 or so years after it was taken, it somehow speaks of redemption.

In rereading the last sentence, I paused to consider why I had used the word *redemption*. It felt right, but I wasn't quite clear in my own mind just why. Anyway, the sentence stood, and a day or two later I received an email that was both odd and welcomed. A McCloskey cousin I had met just once sent me an *Ottawa Citizen* newspaper article out of the blue, dated September 19, 1932. My first thought was who—who is not an archivist—has an intact article from that long ago? And more puzzling, it was an article of limited and finite local interest entitled "One Boy Gallantly Goes to Aid of His Comrade."

Apparently, Dad, age 12, and a chum, age 10, had climbed a centre-town convent wall to steal apples. The younger one fell into the yard and was attacked by a police dog, with my dad gallantly (an old-fashioned word if ever there was one) dropping to the ground to fight off the dog so his chum could escape. The article then proceeded to list the number of stitches—Dad, 21; chum, just 12, but with a bone exposed—time spent in hospital, and the fate of the dog. Apart from chronicling a bygone era of journalism, it does speak to an articulation of record that both terrifies and inspires. What if what we do, that is everything we do, has meaning and is not forgotten? What if even our ruminations of regret and longing to have done better are recorded and await our assessment of self, our bewildered look in the mirror as we meet who we are with recognition for the first time? My use of the word *redemption* came into focus.

Looking at that photo of Dad recently I was reminded of an incident that occurred when I was 15. We did not need parental prompting, lessons, organized leagues, or health promotion lectures to exercise and play sports. We moved, came home for meals, and left quickly to move again. Right after dinner one early summer evening, I grabbed one of our family's much used communal bikes and raced off to join the guys for our daily football game. As I cut through a parking lot my wheel hit a low innocuous cut curb, which I had done innumerable times before.

Though I only found this out later, my front wheel flew off, and I catapulted over the handlebars and hit the pavement head and face first. It had happened so quickly and so spectacularly that I had not had time to get an arm or hand in front of me. I staggered to my feet, confused and aimless, until a lady stopped her car and offered to drive me home. Apparently, I had the wherewithal to remember where I lived, though I could not prevent myself from bleeding all over her car.

I was a mess. Many stitches needed, one tooth broken off, front tooth loose and cracked, and my face a large continuous scab. In the emergency ward waiting for stitches, even my unemotive dad grimaced at the sight of me. One of my older brothers and his friend, a local tough who never gave me the time of day, dropped by and said by way of support, "Chicks dig guys with scars."

In time, the scars faded and the incident was forgotten.

But, then again, maybe not. As I write this, I am dreading dental surgery, which may be why I started thinking about the bike incident again. The front tooth I cracked that day was okay for about 25 years before requiring a root canal. But the root canal could not address that the dead tooth had cracked where it attaches to my jaw bone, and so it will have to come out. The cracked bone will require a bone graft and that I wear a removable fake front tooth for six months until a permanent replacement can be installed. No big deal, but irritating, and something I have been putting off for months. Not an interesting or inspiring topic. In fact, it felt like a weird trivial and distracting rumination.

It is no coincidence that I ended up as an orderly on the spinal cord unit—my dad's isolation and immobility drew me to the work, to the people. I was moved by immobility. It also scared the hell out of me. All of which may be why I had this thought as I thought about my cracked tooth. I now know how Peter and many other guys became quadriplegics, and for many, their accident was no more likely to cause quadriplegia than my bike incident. So why not me? Arbitrary luck of the draw? Something I did, something they did, in a previous life? I don't think so.

Parenthetically, yesterday over coffee and while still wondering why I was spared, I reminded Mike Nemesvary of his answer to the inevitable *why me* question that follows upon personal tragedy. This time he upped the ante, deadpanning, "Why *not* me?" And being serious, he continued, "I never asked why me, but why not me seemed logical. Stuff happens in life; I was a risk-taker and it happened to me. I woke up and dealt with it." The thing about Mike is this: you can marvel at him, you can be impressed by him or question why it has to be his way again, but you cannot doubt him. He woke up to quadriplegia, never asked *why me*? but thought *why not me*? Know a guy for 30 years, bask in his many accomplishments, and the next time you meet to shoot the breeze, he levels you with astonishment. Never lose the ability to surprise. Never lose the ability to be surprised, especially by those you know best.

Mike shamefully reminds me that we don't feel or express gratitude enough, not enough for what we have, barely registering for what we have not had to endure. My bike accident could have broken my spine instead of my tooth, and if the difference between tooth and neck involves sacrifice, it is fair to say that nobody is going to offer to take on quadriplegia for me. Maybe achieving our higher self is the realization of soul, and perhaps my good luck is really the sacrifice of soul from another source for either the individual or collective bank of human need. Nothing could explain such madness except love, which may have far greater meaning than the cliché version we have grown accustomed to.

My dad was not only what happened to him. Real character, one's higher self, exists in how one conducts oneself within the parameters of managing the vicissitudes of a life we never planned for and cannot even reasonably handle. Except that many, many people do just that. I will always be haunted by the image of my dad, age 15, caressing the camera with his knowing eye, confident of just who he is in the holy moment. That moment lives still. There is a photo of my dad.

• • •

I never did learn to pray. Properly. I faked it as a kid those tedious times when Mom and Dad insisted that the entire family get on its knees to recite the rosary. I never could focus my mind, see the purpose or point of it all. We were brought up to appreciate the vague ritualized and rigid articulation of the soul and not to give in to the passionate and haunting inarticulate speech of the heart. The expected negation of self contributed to a sense of separation between heart and soul, and only later did we suspect that they were reconcilable parts; they were the same.

And then, caught up in the business and distraction of the world, decades pass, people pass, and the inexplicable nature and reason for life remains. Still, many people claim to be comfortable not knowing an ultimate or any purpose outside of personal goals. Modern folks tend to be less inclined than all previous generations (which is the basis for the rise of atheism, after all) to agonize over what role we humans could play in the big unfolding of the universe. We are strangely and disingenuously suspended between our narcissistic self-importance and a sense of our insignificance as a speck of meaningless matter in a material world, in the colossus of the universe, within an infinity of multiverses. Not a cozy image but understandable material-world thinking, since it is only the inward gaze that allows us to distract from fully comprehending our insignificance and purposelessness, which would surely lead to madness. We shrug and say, "That's life" as solace against feeling, defence against despair, rationale for not thinking too deeply.

The great dumbing down of our or any age may temporarily feel good but ultimately will not comfort us. There is irony in the pursuit of comfort as a virtue. Beneath our epic distraction is embryonic despair, the silent scream to release pain, love, loneliness, loss, compassion, the inarticulate speech of the heart. For all we invest in avoidance, the need to release is part of our human essence and will not go away. In fact, we experience more pain, more loneliness for expressing less; less is more, but not in a good way. The unavoidable truth—that we spend a lifetime avoiding—is that the inarticulate speech of the heart is yearning to be known and to know others. It is art. It is beauty. It is reaching out. It is turning back one step and dropping coins into the hat. It is the revelation of a face you've seen a thousand times but whose essence you had missed until this moment. It is reminding ourselves that intending is not doing, and our higher self is just that, always higher, and since we can do better, must do better, there are no laurels to rest upon.

I was never satisfied winning a race or achieving a personal best time. Cara says I never take time to reflect on something I've done well, and she's right. Maybe I should, but I can't. Whatever is done is done, and I always want to do better, am deeply suspicious of self-satisfaction, am determined to translate intention into action. Satisfaction for successfully translating intention into action is not action. Make sense? A human perversity maybe, but not complacency, at least not that. And as for when I do badly, react or act from my lower self, recrimination, even if not immediate, haunts my dreams, stirring wakefulness into false dawn. No doubt the curse of Irish Catholic conscience and the resultant fog of guilt.

We disparage guilt today and have made its opposite a virtue—the perpetual expression of self in a guilt-free world is considered a life well lived. If not for the fact that in the safest, freest, most affluent time in history people are increasingly anxious, depressed, lonely, and lost, I might agree. It ain't working out, because uncool as it may be to utilize conscience and act on guilt, it as a precursor to compassion is our saving grace; it is where we exit self, have the potential to intersect with another's consciousness, and with a modicum of understanding, it is where the possibility of elevating from our solitary consciousness to living *in* consciousness exists.

Pangs of conscience—good and bad, and guilt—not necessarily good or bad, pervade my thoughts, dreams, and memories, rerunning, ruminating on, the daily film, showing me how I could have done better, should have connected more, had I not chosen to exist in a singular, solitary state. Seems harsh, I know, but life is harsh, complacency creates an illusion, and deliberate efforts are the only way to exist *in* consciousness, to make a connection between locked-in lives and lonely souls.

We need compassion, we need movement, always, because we never actually get over grief, we never actually stop loving those we have loved, and if our life's purpose is determined by whomever God places in our path, then we can never be fully distant from another's pain. The concept that a parent can only be as happy as the unhappiest of his children ultimately extends to the clutter, debris, and singular beauty of any human being on our path. And, to overwhelm with the astonishing nature of potential for purpose, all of humanity is in our path.

With apologies to my mom, I never learned to formally pray, but in consideration of my cluttered path, my pre-dawn awakenings have morphed into a kind of desperate prayer. In the 1993 film *Shadowlands*, Anthony Hopkins plays writer C. S. Lewis, who meets and marries American poet Joy Davidman. The central feature of their magnificent love is that she allows the great C. S. Lewis to articulate, for the first time in his life, the inarticulate speech of his heart. It is his exiting the shadowlands of his repressive heart that the film is named for. But he becomes inconsolable after her unexpected death, so his friend offers a trite, obtuse piece of advice: "Why don't you pray?" To which the normally controlled Lewis erupts that prayer, desperate and pervasive, is all he is able to do, every minute of every day; that prayer oozes out of every pore, to the point of insanity without relief. He cannot but pray because that is where living, loving, and grieving lead us. And it occurred to me that without the insulation of distraction and denial—in short, modernity—a crisis of articulation is what, in a very real sense, life amounts to. Perhaps prayer—consciousness infused with intention—is our means to address the "gap" between inarticulate speech and what, of the heart, remains unspoken. Gibran stated, "Between what is said and not meant, and what is meant and not said, most of love is lost."

Many, perhaps most, have moved on from desperate and archaic rituals of the past. Though we think we have arrived at a superior epoch of time from which we know far more than previous generations—never mind that we have lost the capacity to differentiate between wisdom and data—we understand less for knowing more. Still, some few of us subversives seek refuge in time. Maybe where we are in time doesn't matter because time doesn't matter, at least in the way we have ordered ourselves around the certainty of sequential, linear time. I can't help thinking that *in* consciousness, time is not linear and past but perpetual and here for now and all time. And if we are not past time, we continue to be responsible for what we do in time, for all time—a sort of accountability on steroids, wherein everyone placed along our path, everyone we have helped and hindered, contributes to revelation, is our ever-present personal God.

I am haunted by 10,000 highly personal thoughts and images that I am powerless to do anything about, even if I wanted to do anything, which I do not. The inarticulate speech of my pathetic heart rages, often powerless to express or else expressing without being heard, plagued by conscience and compassion for people long since gone, on my path here and now, or still to come. I am haunted and pray because I cannot reconcile myself to modernity's brute force interpretation of life, because love and compassion cannot simply vanish because I must.

Dreams, nightmares, depressed thoughts, and inspired moments return, visiting Chris's expression as he pounds his lifeless legs that will not feel or walk again; the moment that Gord's vision disappears and he is left feeling his way out of a Welsh pub and back to his lonely room; the ecstasy of Janice's laugh; my sense of extraordinary staring down at Paul's ordinary cursive written note; my material-world impulse to impose ordinary on extraordinary as the stereo lights up and surround sounds fill the house; recognizing perfection in my daughters and my daughters' daughters, that they cannot see that I cannot unsee; those seconds during the marathon, passing the other Paul, who has waited for hours; Terry's moment of letting go of his girlfriend and his former life; Mike's 40 hours of loneliness, not knowing if anyone will come; Dad's misadventure at sea during the war that resulted in his broken back and diminished dreams, which he could not articulate, for which a pattern of inarticulation descended upon our family; Zigo's exemplary spiritual guidance; Doug's ache to be loved; Peter's question about a personal God, and how I still must find an answer that is not facile, simplistic, or condescending.

For all this and more I cannot help but pray, even if my present prayers are resurrected from lower states, such as anxiety, depression, rumination, and worry. And, of course, there is always guilt and conscience. But whatever emotional cocktail resides in my brain, your brain, everyone's brain, when there is love and compassion, we are all humble supplicants, it is painfully personal prayer, and there is hope. From the periphery of *in* consciousness, wrapped up with the cast of characters that populate my crowded path, my personal God is revealed to the extent that my prayers are personal. At which point everything is personal. A personal God exists wherever there is a wounded psyche and an open heart.

ACKNOWLEDGEMENTS

We didn't make ourselves. We didn't create what we see around us. My awareness of self, and to the extent I can pierce the inarticulate heart of another, is not from knowing. Our lacking is not ignorance but insight into the infamous "I think therefore I am" as a precursor to knowing that you, all seven billion of you, are there.

Writers don't actually go to South Seas islands to write alone. All creative work requires context and content. *If not for the grace of God* lets us pick up the pen, and *whomever God places along our path* is the stuff of narrative dreams that allows us to soar. The people who lend you reasons to write aren't necessarily connected to it. Writing for me is love made real. Seems trite but is true. The following people have contributed to this book, and some even know it.

Amanda and Dean Mellway

Paul, Donald, and Jerome Menton and Margaret (Manery) Menton

Cara Lipsett

Daughters Shannon, Kristen, and Caitlin McCloskey; granddaughters Pearl, Penny, and Georgia

Susan Prosser and John Meissner

Dale and Richard Taylor

Linda and Paddy Stewart

Marina Hofman Willard and Larry Willard

Chris and Heather Barrett

John Weston

Donna McCloskey

Patrick McCloskey

Tony Shaw

Mike Nemesvary

Don Cumming

Somei Tam

Melanie Rock and Daryl Rock

Tanis Browning-Shelp

Dawn Brown
Max Finkelstein
Doug Macklem
Peter McGrath
Zigo (thinks he's people, so close enough)

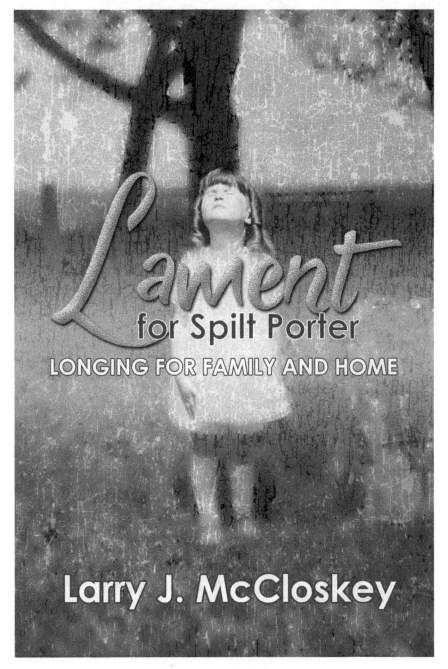

Lament
for Spilt Porter
LONGING FOR FAMILY AND HOME

Larry J. McCloskey

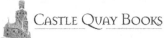

CASTLE QUAY BOOKS

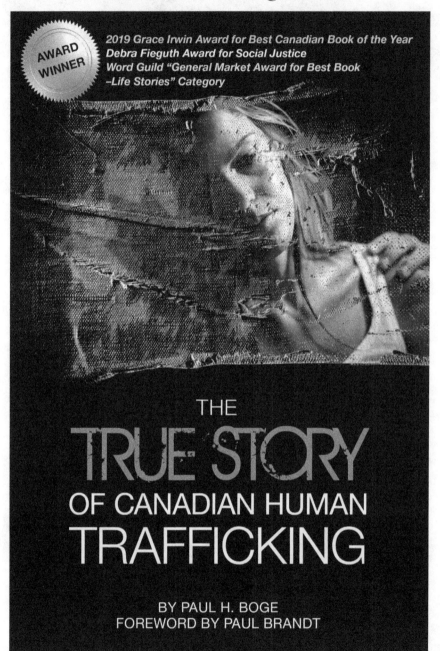

AWARD WINNER

2019 Grace Irwin Award for Best Canadian Book of the Year
Debra Fieguth Award for Social Justice
Word Guild "General Market Award for Best Book
–Life Stories" Category

THE
TRUE STORY
OF CANADIAN HUMAN
TRAFFICKING

BY PAUL H. BOGE
FOREWORD BY PAUL BRANDT

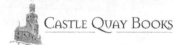

CASTLE QUAY BOOKS

RISEN FROM PRISON

BEYOND MY WILDEST IMAGINATION

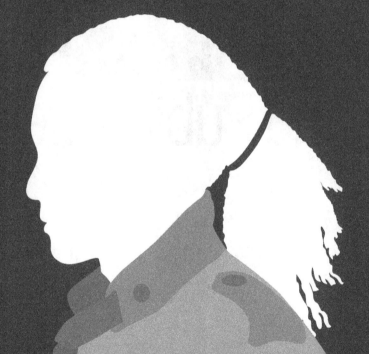

BOSCO H.C. POON

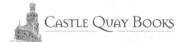

CASTLE QUAY BOOKS

Faith, LEADERSHIP and Public Life

Leadership Lessons from Moses to Jesus

Preston Manning

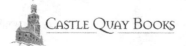

CASTLE QUAY BOOKS

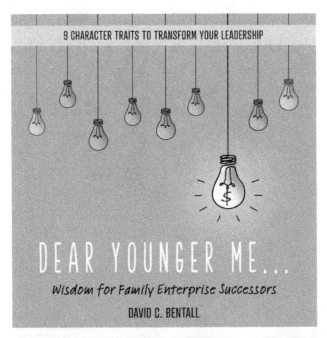

9 CHARACTER TRAITS TO TRANSFORM YOUR LEADERSHIP

DEAR YOUNGER ME...

Wisdom for Family Enterprise Successors

DAVID C. BENTALL

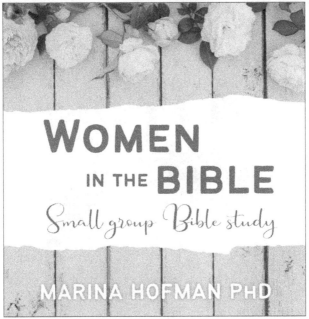

WOMEN
IN THE BIBLE
Small group Bible study

MARINA HOFMAN PhD

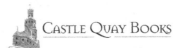

CASTLE QUAY BOOKS

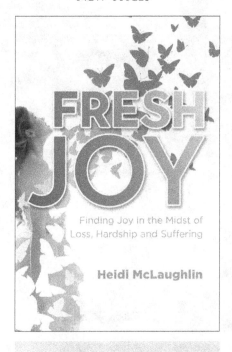

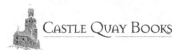

CASTLE QUAY BOOKS

CPSIA information can be obtained
at www.ICGtesting.com
Printed in the USA
LVHW011905190721
693094LV00003B/593

9 781988 928395